The Ultimate Diabetic Diet Collection for Busy People

Quick and Delicious Recipes to Enjoy Your Diet and Make Healthy Meals

Lesly Mclean

Table of contents

Scallion Sandwich

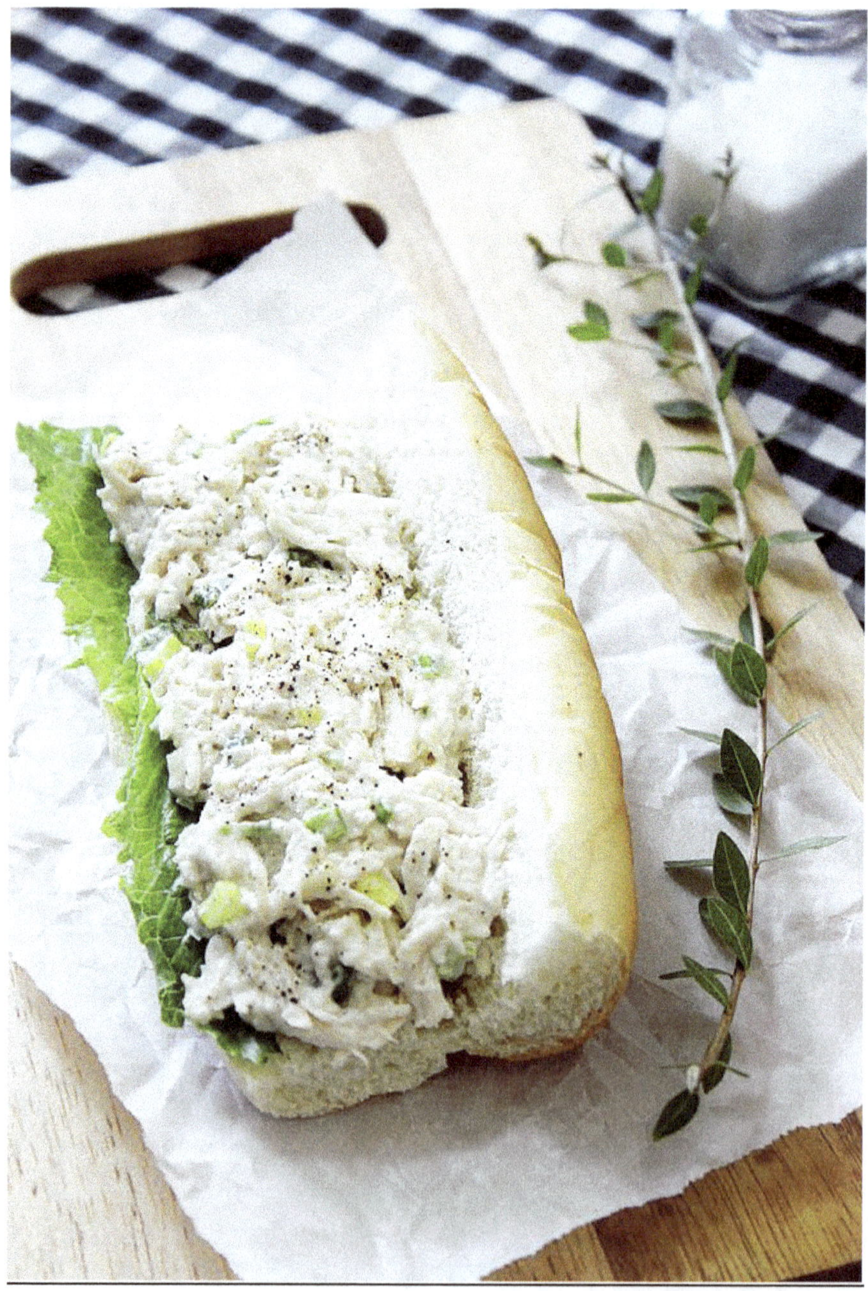

Preparation Time : 10 minutes

Cooking Time : 10 minutes

Servings : 1

Ingredients :

- 2 slices wheat bread
- 2 teaspoons butter, low fat
- 2 scallions, sliced thinly
- 1 tablespoon of parmesan cheese, grated
- 3/4 cup of cheddar cheese, reduced fat, grated

Directions :

1. Preheat the Air fryer to 356 degrees.
2. Spread butter on a slice of bread. Place inside the cooking basket with the butter side facing down.
3. Place cheese and scallions on top. Spread the rest of the butter on the other slice of bread Put it on top of the sandwich and sprinkle with parmesan cheese.
4. Cook for 10 minutes.

Nutrition : Calorie: 154; Carbohydrate: 9g; Fat: 2.5g; Protein: 8.6g; Fiber: 2.4g

Lean Lamb and Turkey Meatballs with Yogurt

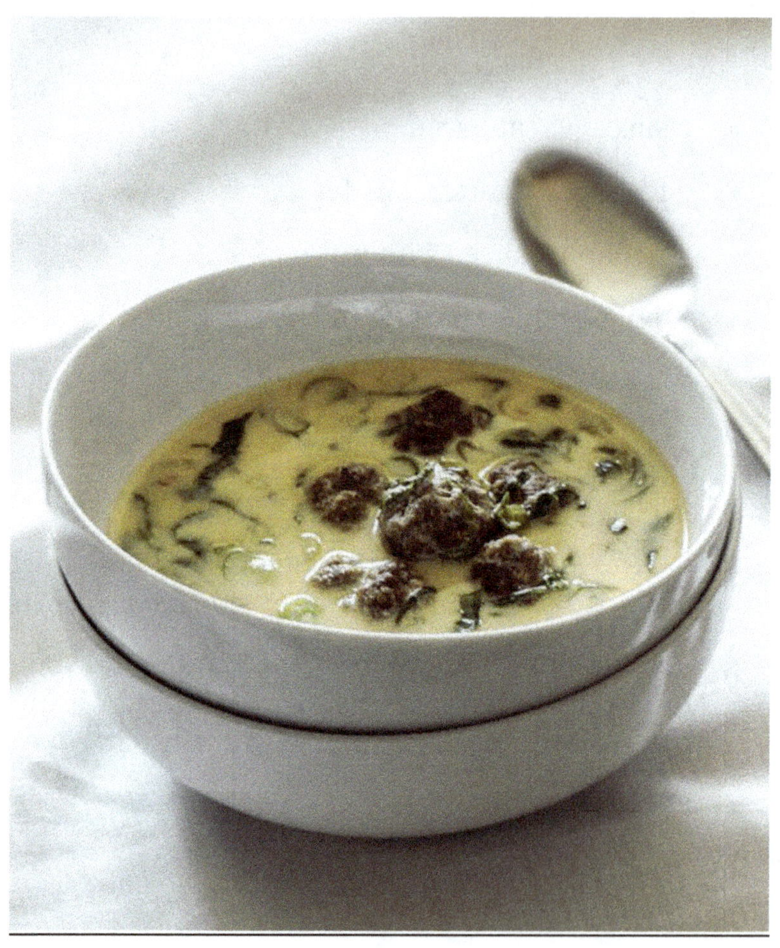

Preparation Time : 10 minutes

Servings : 4

Cooking Time : 8 minutes

Ingredients :

- 1 egg white

- 4 ounces ground lean turkey

- 1 pound of ground lean lamb

- 1 teaspoon each of cayenne pepper, ground coriander, red chili pastes, salt, and ground cumin

- 2 garlic cloves, minced

- 1 1/2 tablespoons parsley, chopped

- 1 tablespoon mint, chopped

- 1/4 cup of olive oil

For the yogurt

- 2 tablespoons of buttermilk

- 1 garlic clove, minced

- 1/4 cup mint, chopped

- 1/2 cup of Greek yogurt, non-fat

- Salt to taste

Directions :

1. Set the Air Fryer to 390 degrees.

2. Mix all the ingredients for the meatballs in a bowl. Roll and mold them into golf-size round pieces. Arrange in the cooking basket. Cook for 8 minutes.

3. While waiting, combine all the ingredients for the mint yogurt in a bowl. Mix well.

4. Serve the meatballs with the mint yogurt. Top with olives and fresh mint.

Nutrition : Calorie: 154; Carbohydrate: 9g; Fat: 2.5g; Protein: 8.6g; Fiber: 2.4g

Air Fried Section and Tomato

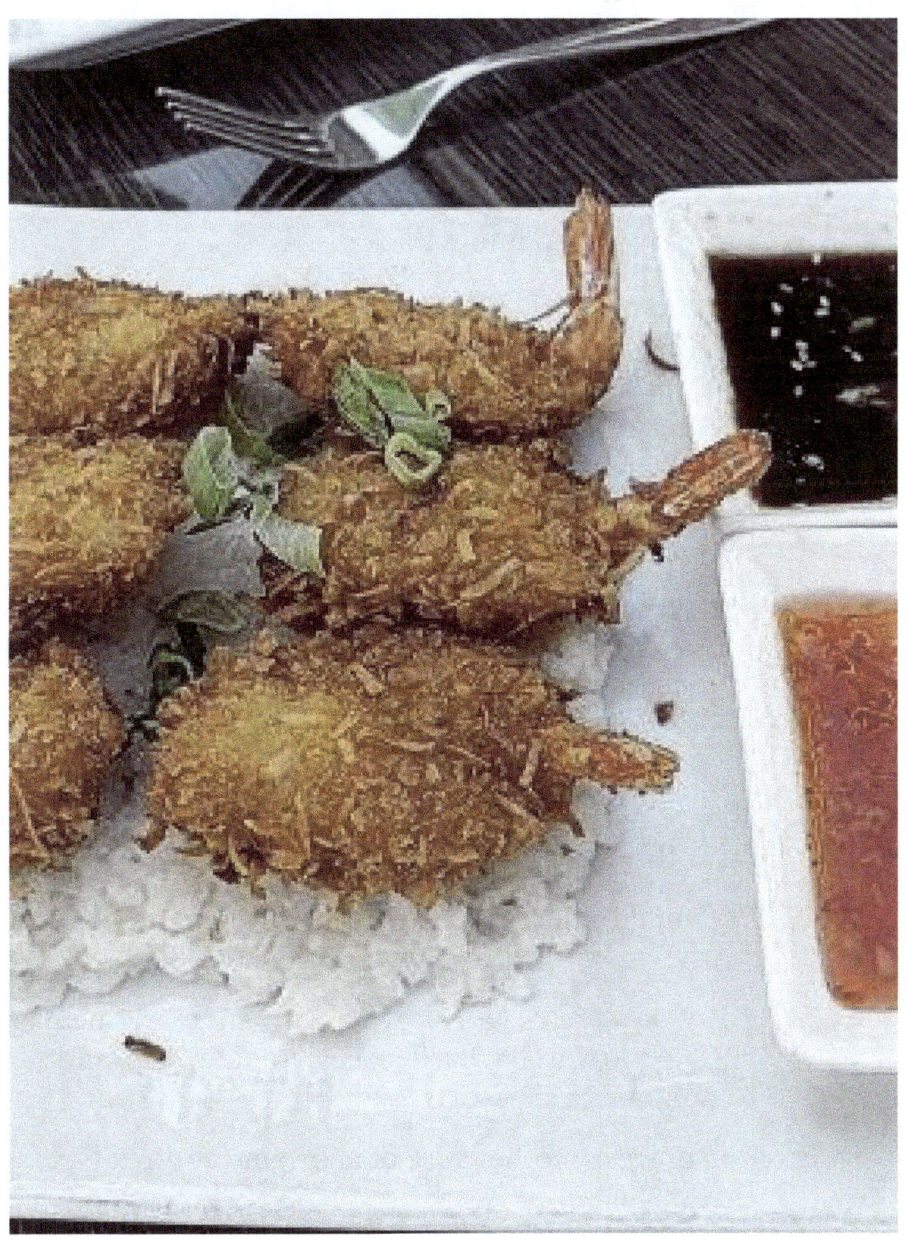

<u>*Preparation Time*</u> : 10 minutes

<u>*Cooking Time*</u> : 5 minutes

<u>*Servings*</u> : 2

<u>*Ingredients*</u> :

- 1 aubergine, sliced thickly into 4 disks
- 1 tomato, sliced into 2 thick disks
- 2 tsp. feta cheese, reduced fat
- 2 fresh basil leaves, minced
- 2 balls, small buffalo mozzarella, reduced fat, roughly torn
- Pinch of salt
- Pinch of black pepper

<u>*Directions*</u> :

1. Preheat Air Fryer to 330 degrees F.

2. Spray small amount of oil into the Air fryer basket. Fry aubergine slices for 5 minutes or until golden brown on both sides. Transfer to a plate.

3. Fry tomato slices in batches for 5 minutes or until seared on both sides.

4. To serve, stack salad starting with an aborigine base, buffalo mozzarella, basil leaves, tomato slice, and 1/2-teaspoon feta cheese.

5. Top of with another slice of aborigine and 1/2 tsp. feta cheese. Serve.

<u>*Nutrition*</u> : Calorie: 140.3; Carbohydrate: 26.6; Fat: 3.4g; Protein: 4.2g; Fiber: 7.3g

Cheesy Salmon Fillets

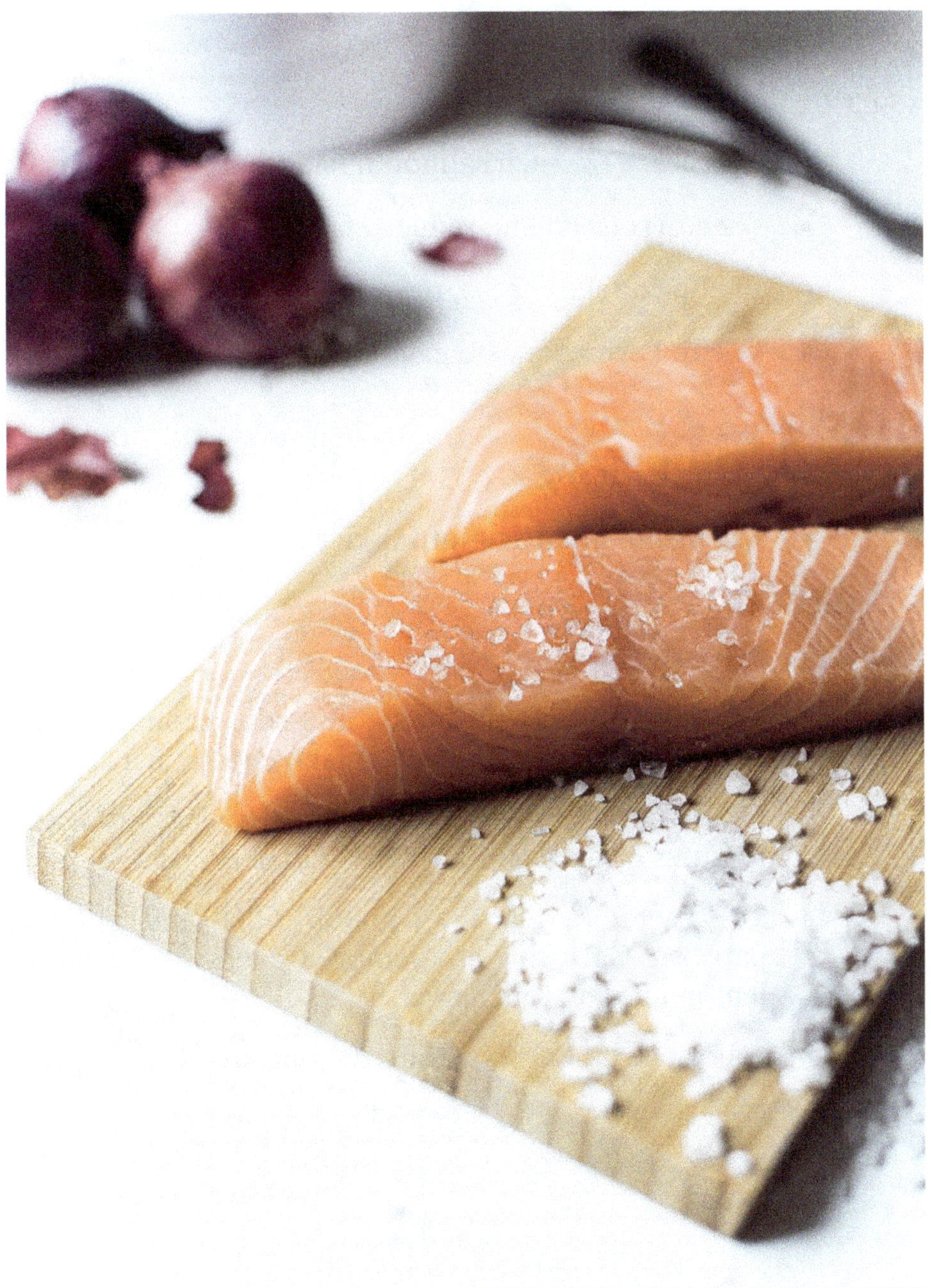

Preparation Time : 15 minutes

Cooking Time : 20 minutes

Servings : 2-3

Ingredients : For the salmon fillets

- 2 pieces, 4 oz. each salmon fillets, choose even cuts

- 1/2 cup sour cream, reduced fat

- ¼ cup cottage cheese, reduced fat

- ¼ cup Parmigiano-Reggiano cheese, freshly grated

Garnish:

- Spanish paprika

- 1/2-piece lemon, cut into wedges

Directions :

1. Preheat Air Fryer to 330 degrees F.

2. To make the salmon fillets, mix sour cream, cottage cheese, and Parmigiano-Reggiano cheese in a bowl.

3. Layer salmon fillets in the Air fryer basket. Fry for 20 minutes or until cheese turns golden brown.

4. To assemble, place a salmon fillet and sprinkle paprika. Garnish with lemon wedges and squeeze lemon juice on top. Serve.

Nutrition : Calorie: 274; Carbohydrate: 1g; Fat: 19g; Protein: 24g; Fiber: 0.5g

Salmon with Asparagus

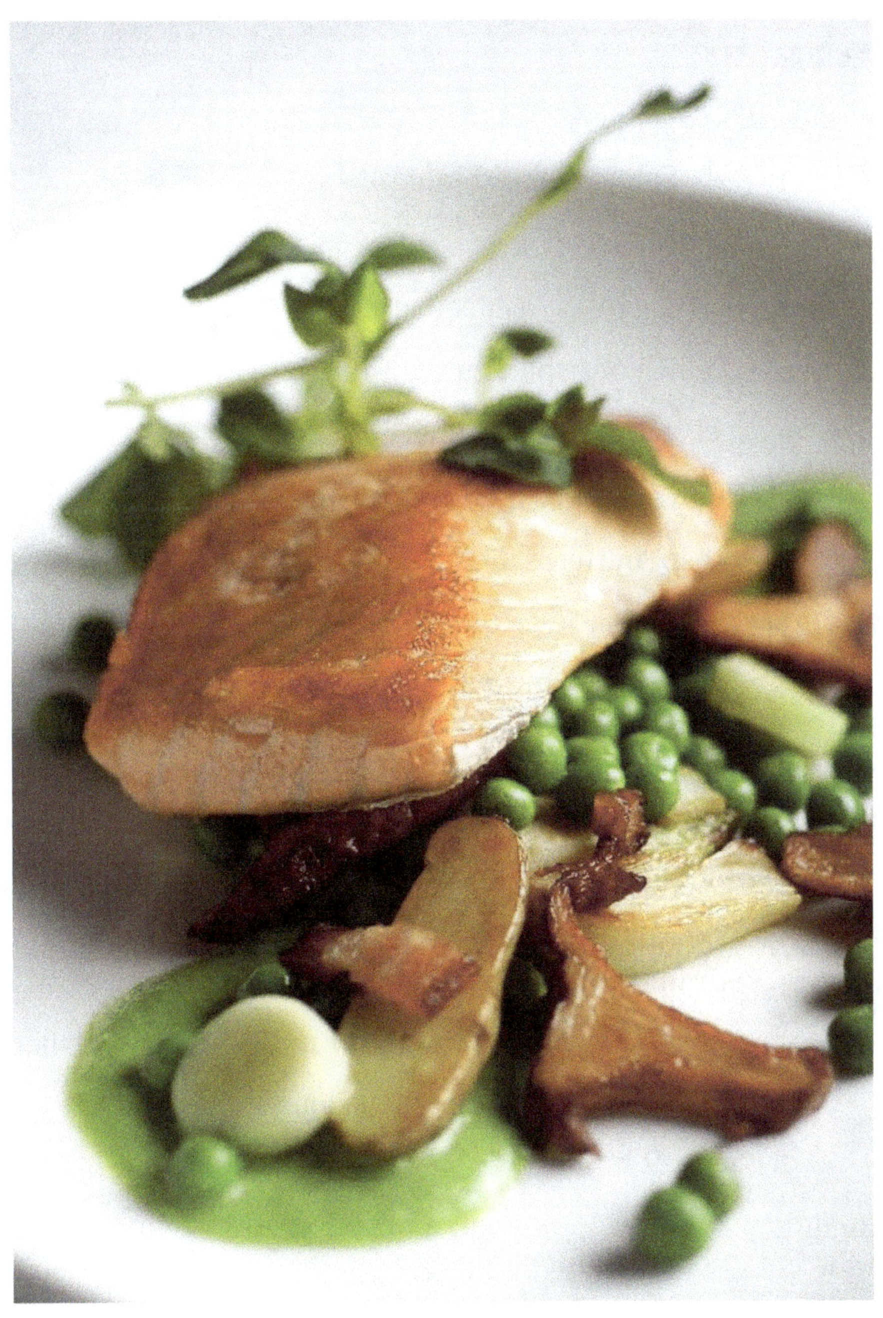

Preparation Time : 5 Minutes

Cooking Time : 10 Minutes

Servings : 3

Ingredients :

- 1 lb. Salmon, sliced into fillets
- 1 tbsp. Olive Oil
- Salt & Pepper, as needed
- 1 bunch of Asparagus, trimmed
- 2 cloves of Garlic, minced
- Zest & Juice of 1/2 Lemon
- 1 tbsp. Butter, salted

Directions :

1. Spoon in the butter and olive oil into a large pan and heat it over medium-high heat.
2. Once it becomes hot, place the salmon and season it with salt and pepper.
3. Cook for 4 minutes per side and then cook the other side.
4. Stir in the garlic and lemon zest to it.
5. Cook for further 2 minutes or until slightly browned.
6. Off the heat and squeeze the lemon juice over it.
7. Serve it hot.

Nutrition : Calories: 409Kcal; Carbohydrates: 2.7g; Proteins: 32.8g; Fat: 28.8g; Sodium: 497mg

Shrimp in Garlic Butter

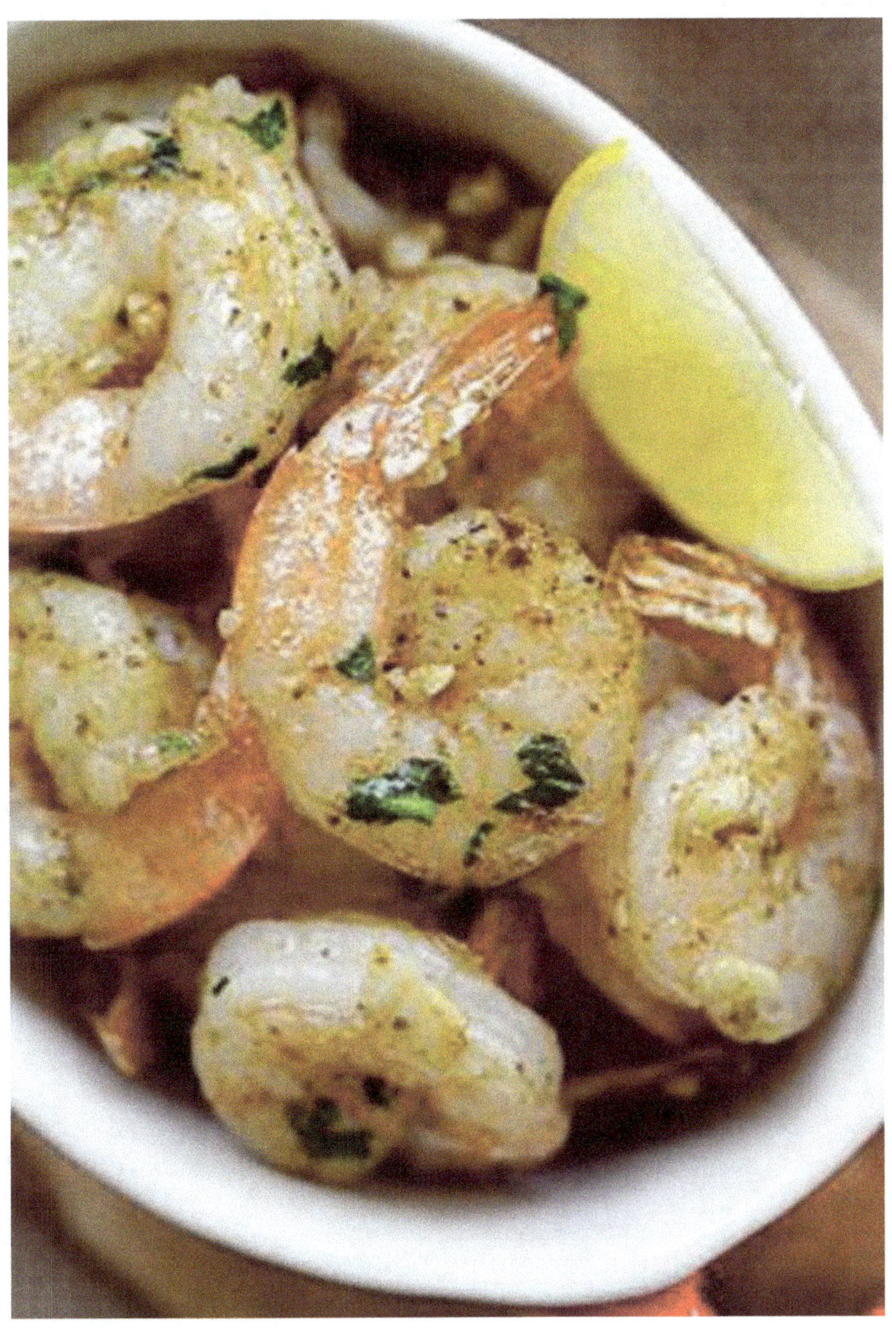

<u>*Preparation Time*</u> : 5 Minutes

<u>*Cooking Time*</u> : 20 Minutes

<u>*Servings*</u> : 4

<u>*Ingredients*</u> :

- 1 lb. Shrimp, peeled & deveined
- ¼ tsp. Red Pepper Flakes
- 6 tbsp. Butter, divided
- 1/2 cup Chicken Stock
- Salt & Pepper, as needed
- 2 tbsp. Parsley, minced
- 5 cloves of Garlic, minced
- 2 tbsp. Lemon Juice

<u>*Directions*</u> :

1. Heat a large bottomed skillet over medium-high heat.
2. Spoon in two tablespoons of the butter and melt it. Add the shrimp.
3. Season it with salt and pepper. Sear for 4 minutes or until shrimp gets cooked.
4. Transfer the shrimp to a plate and stir in the garlic.
5. Sauté for 30 seconds or until aromatic.
6. Pour the chicken stock and whisk it well. Allow it to simmer for 5 to 10 minutes or until it has reduced to half.
7. Spoon the remaining butter, red pepper, and lemon juice to the sauce. Mix.

8. Continue cooking for another 2 minutes.

9. Take off the pan from the heat and add the cooked shrimp to it.

10. Garnish with parsley and transfer to the serving bowl.

11. Enjoy.

Nutrition : Calories: 307Kcal; Carbohydrates: 3g; Proteins: 27g; Fat: 20g; Sodium: 522mg

Cobb Salad
Keto & Under 30 Minutes

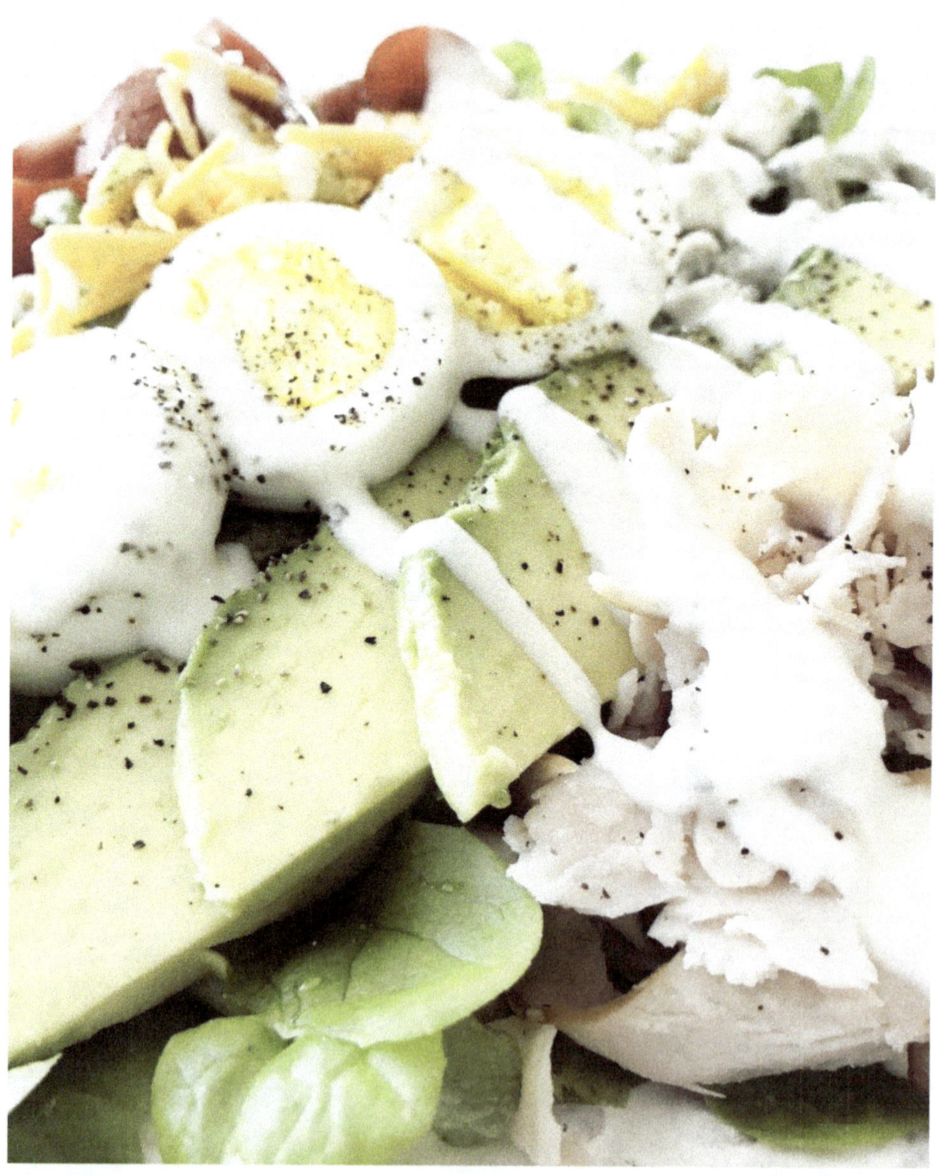

Preparation Time : 5 Minutes

Cooking Time : 5 Minutes

Servings : 1

Ingredients :

- 4 Cherry Tomatoes, chopped
- ¼ cup Bacon, cooked & crumbled
- 1/2 of 1 Avocado, chopped
- 2 oz. Chicken Breast, shredded
- 1 Egg, hardboiled
- 2 cups Mixed Green salad
- 1 oz. Feta Cheese, crumbled

Directions :

1. Toss all the ingredients for the Cobb salad in a large mixing bowl and toss well.
2. Serve and enjoy it.

Nutrition : Calories: 307KcalC; arbohydrates: 3g; Proteins: 27g; Fat: 20g; Sodium: 522mg

Seared Tuna Steak

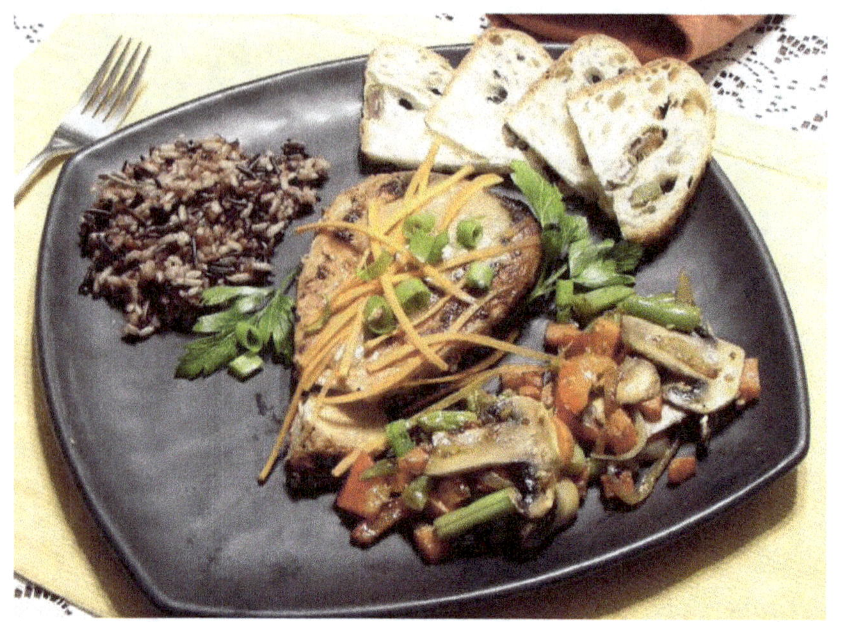

Preparation Time : 10 Minutes

Cooking Time : 10 Minutes

Serving Size : 2

Ingredients :

- 1 tsp. Sesame Seeds
- 1 tbsp. Sesame Oil
- 2 tbsp. Soya Sauce
- Salt & Pepper, to taste
- 2 × 6 oz. Ahi Tuna Steaks

Directions :

1. Seasoning the tuna steaks with salt and pepper. Keep it aside on a shallow bowl.
2. In another bowl, mix soya sauce and sesame oil.
3. pour the sauce over the salmon and coat them generously with the sauce.
4. Keep it aside for 10 to 15 minutes and then heat a large skillet over medium heat.
5. Once hot, keep the tuna steaks and cook them for 3 minutes or until seared underneath.
6. Flip the fillets and cook them for a further 3 minutes.
7. Transfer the seared tuna steaks to the serving plate and slice them into 1/2-inch slices. Top with sesame seeds.

Nutrition : Calories: 255Kcal; Fat: 9g; Carbohydrates: 1g; Proteins: 40.5g; Sodium: 293mg

Beef Chili

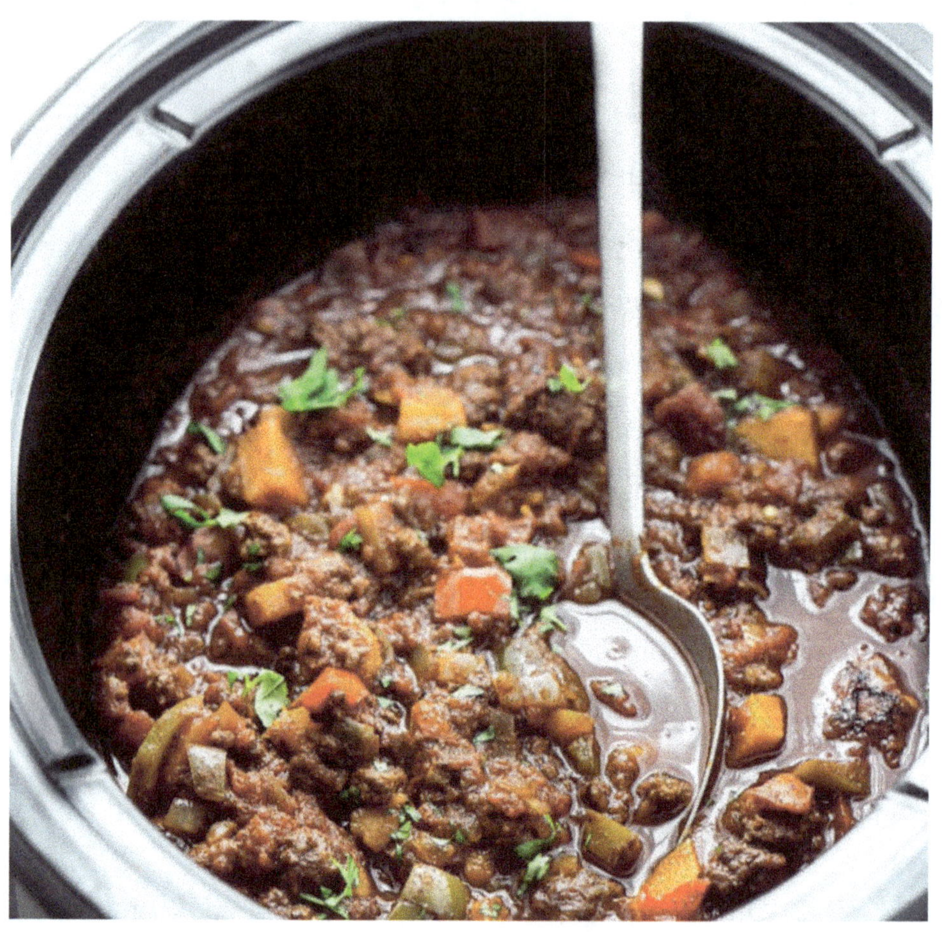

Preparation Time : 10 Minutes

Cooking Time : 20 Minutes

Serving Size : 4

Ingredients :

- 1/2 tsp. Garlic Powder
- 1 tsp. Coriander, grounded
- 1 lb. Beef, grounded
- 1/2 tsp. Sea Salt
- 1/2 tsp. Cayenne Pepper
- 1 tsp. Cumin, grounded
- 1/2 tsp. Pepper, grounded
- 1/2 cup Salsa, low-carb & no-sugar

Directions :

1. Heat a large-sized pan over medium-high heat and cook the beef in it until browned.
2. Stir in all the spices and cook them for 7 minutes or until everything is combined.
3. When the beef gets cooked, spoon in the salsa.
4. Bring the mixture to a simmer and cook for another 8 minutes or until everything comes together.
5. Take it from heat and transfer to a serving bowl.

Nutrition : Calories: 229Kcal; Fat: 10g; Carbohydrates: 2g; Proteins: 33g; Sodium: 675mg

Greek Broccoli Salad

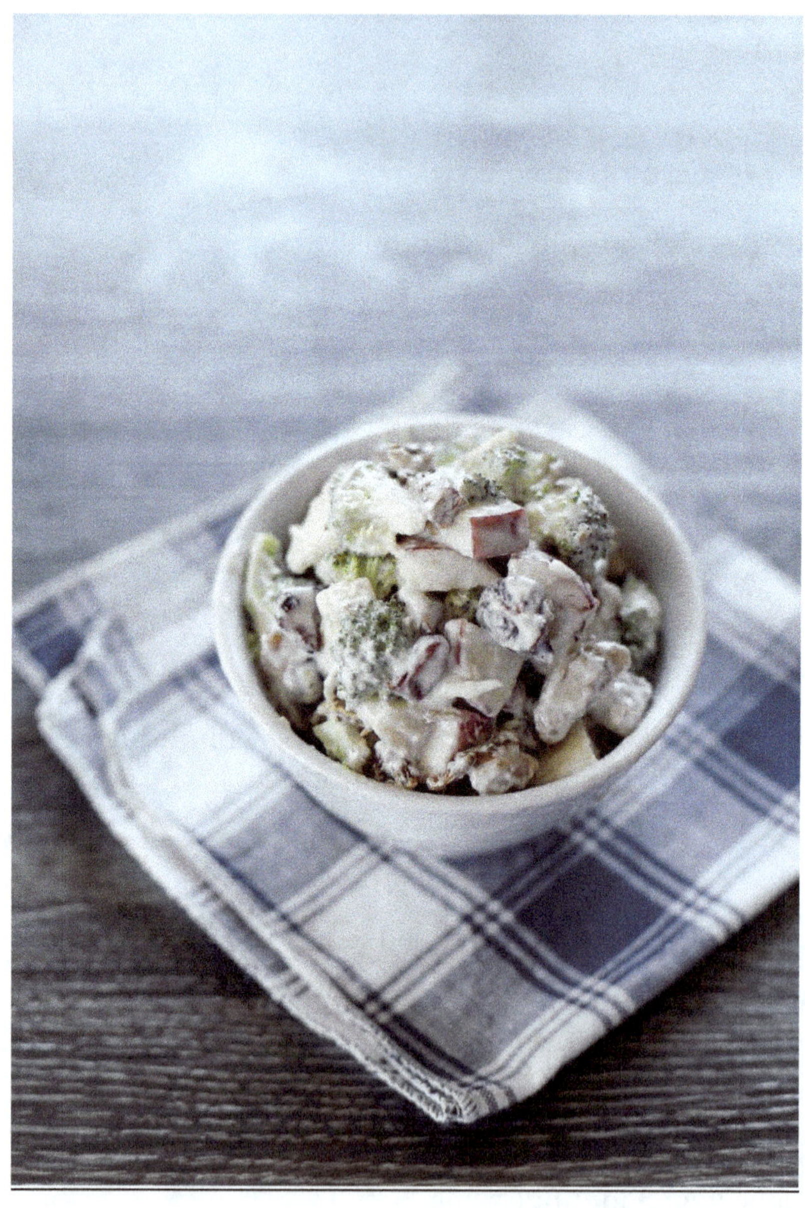

<u>Preparation Time</u> : 10 Minutes

<u>Cooking Time</u> : 15 Minutes

<u>Servings</u> : 4

<u>Ingredients</u> :

- 1 ¼ lb. Broccoli, sliced into small bites
- ¼ cup Almonds, sliced
- 1/3 cup Sun-dried Tomatoes
- ¼ cup Feta Cheese, crumbled
- ¼ cup Red Onion, sliced

For the dressing:

- 1/4 cup Olive Oil
- Dash of Red Pepper Flakes
- 1 Garlic clove, minced
- ¼ tsp. Salt
- 2 tbsp. Lemon Juice
- 1/2 tsp. Dijon Mustard
- 1 tsp. Low Carb Sweetener Syrup
- 1/2 tsp. Oregano, dried

<u>Directions</u> :

1. Mix broccoli, onion, almonds and sun-dried tomatoes in a large mixing bowl.
2. In another small-sized bowl, combine all the dressing ingredients until emulsified.

3. Spoon the dressing over the broccoli salad.

4. Allow the salad to rest for half an hour before serving.

Nutrition : Calories: 272Kcal; Carbohydrates: 11.9g; Proteins: 8g; Fat: 21.6g; Sodium: 321mg

Cheesy Cauliflower Gratin

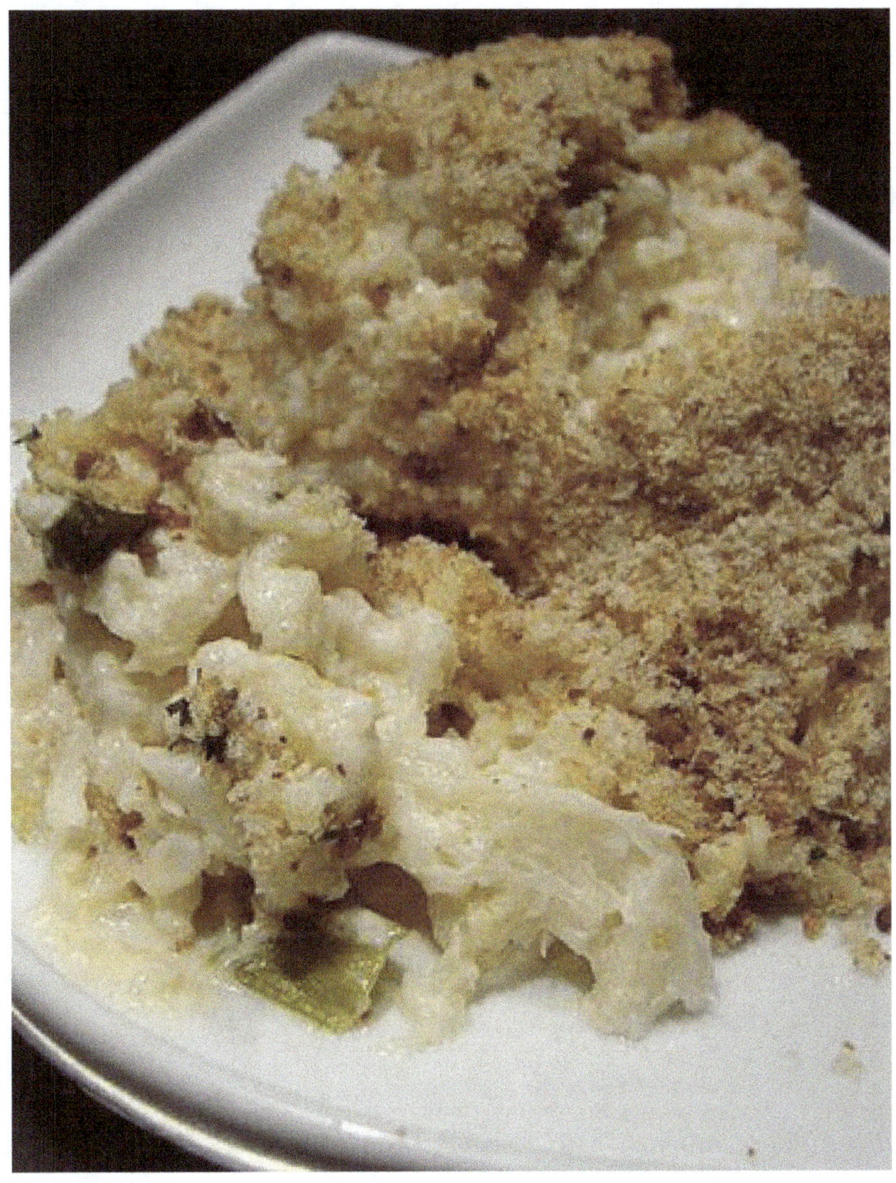

Preparation Time : 5 Minutes

Cooking Time : 25 Minutes

Servings : 6

Ingredients :

- 6 deli slices Pepper Jack Cheese
- 4 cups Cauliflower florets
- Salt and Pepper, as needed
- 4 tbsp. Butter
- 1/3 cup Heavy Whipping Cream

Directions :

1. Mix the cauliflower, cream, butter, salt, and pepper in a safe microwave bowl and combine well.

2. Microwave the cauliflower mixture for 25 minutes on high until it becomes soft and tender.

3. Remove the ingredients from the bowl and mash with the help of a fork.

4. Taste for seasonings and spoon in salt and pepper as required.

5. Arrange the slices of pepper jack cheese on top of the cauliflower mixture and microwave for 3 minutes until the cheese starts melting.

6. Serve warm.

Nutrition : Calories: 421Kcal; Carbohydrates: 3g; Proteins: 19g; Fat: 37g; Sodium: 111mg

Strawberry Spinach Salad

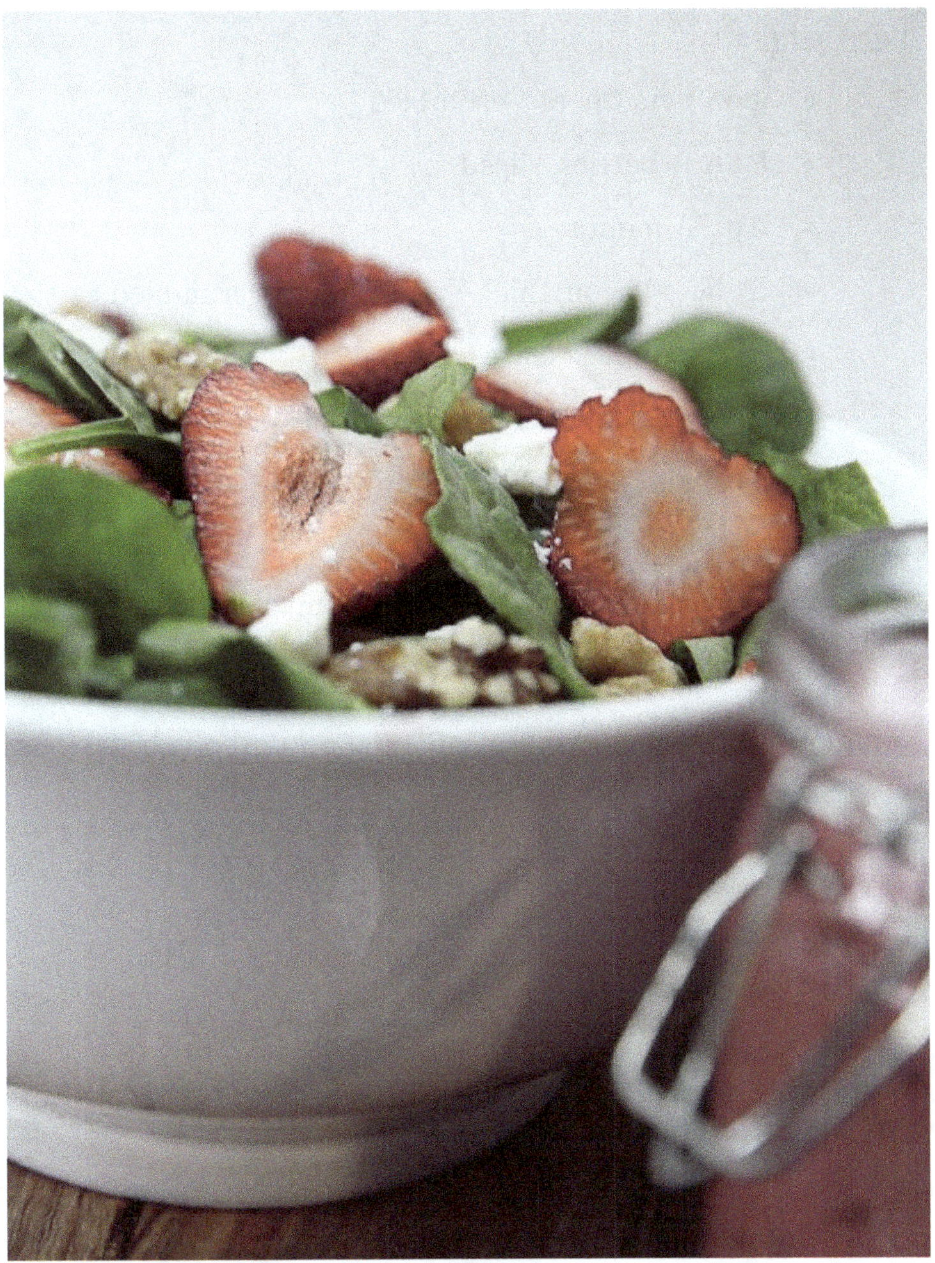

Preparation Time : 5 Minutes

Cooking Time : 10 Minutes

Servings : 4

Ingredients :

- 4 oz. Feta Cheese, crumbled
- 8 Strawberries, sliced
- 2 oz. Almonds
- 6 Slices Bacon, thick-cut, crispy and crumbled
- 10 oz. Spinach leaves, fresh
- 2 Roma Tomatoes, diced
- 2 oz. Red Onion, sliced thinly

Directions :

1. For making this healthy salad, mix all the ingredients needed to make the salad in a large-sized bowl and toss them well.

Nutrition : Calories: 255kcal; Fat: 16g; Carbohydrates: 8g; Proteins: 14g; Sodium: 27mg

Misto Quente

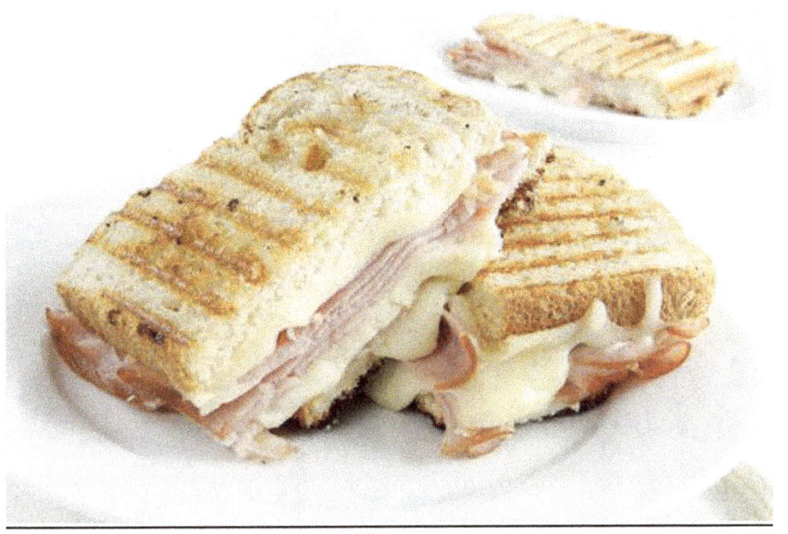

Preparation Time : 5 minutes

Cooking Time : 10 minutes

Servings : 4

Ingredients :

- 4 slices of bread without shell
- 4 slices of turkey breast
- 4 slices of cheese
- 2 tbsp. cream cheese
- 2 spoons of butter

Directions :

1. Preheat the air fryer. Set the timer of 5 minutes and the temperature to 200C.

2. Pass the butter on one side of the slice of bread, and on the other side of the slice, the cream cheese.

3. Mount the sandwiches placing two slices of turkey breast and two slices cheese between the breads, with the cream cheese inside and the side with butter.

4. Place the sandwiches in the basket of the air fryer. Set the timer of the air fryer for 5 minutes and press the power button.

Nutrition : Calories: 340; Fat: 15g; Carbohydrates: 32g; Protein: 15g; Sugar: 0g; Cholesterol: 0mg

Garlic Bread

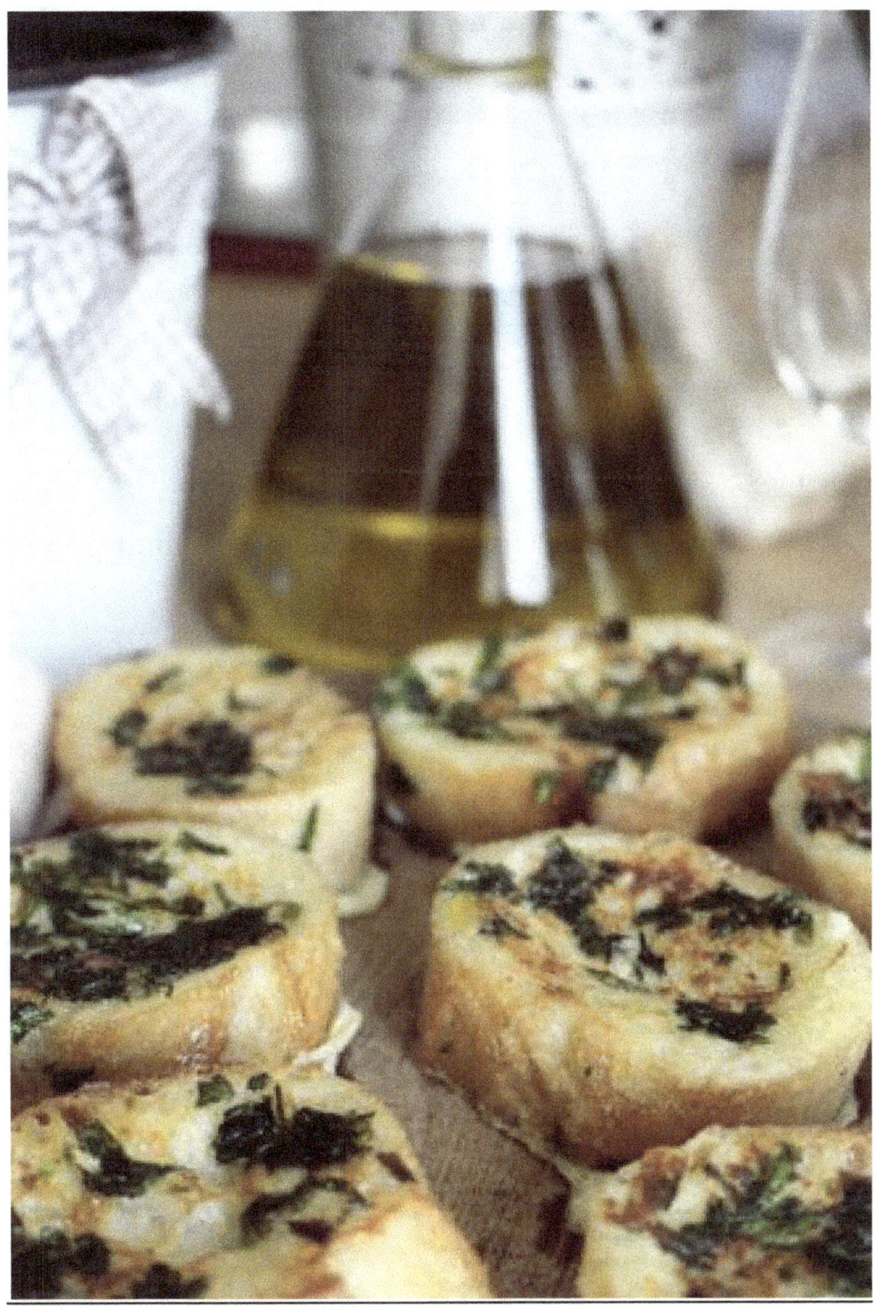

Preparation Time : 10 minutes

Cooking Time : 15 minutes

Servings : 4-5

Ingredients :

- 2 stale French rolls
- 4 tbsp. crushed or crumpled garlic
- 1 cup of mayonnaise
- Powdered grated Parmesan
- 1 tbsp. olive oil

Directions :

1. Preheat the air fryer. Set the time of 5 minutes and the temperature to 2000C.

2. Mix mayonnaise with garlic and set aside.

3. Cut the baguettes into slices, but without separating them completely.

4. Fill the cavities of equals. Brush with olive oil and sprinkle with grated cheese.

5. Place in the basket of the air fryer. Set the timer to 10 minutes, adjust the temperature to 1800C and press the power button.

Nutrition : Calories: 340; Fat: 15g; Carbohydrates: 32g; Protein: 15g Sugar: 0g; Cholesterol: 0mg

Bruschetta

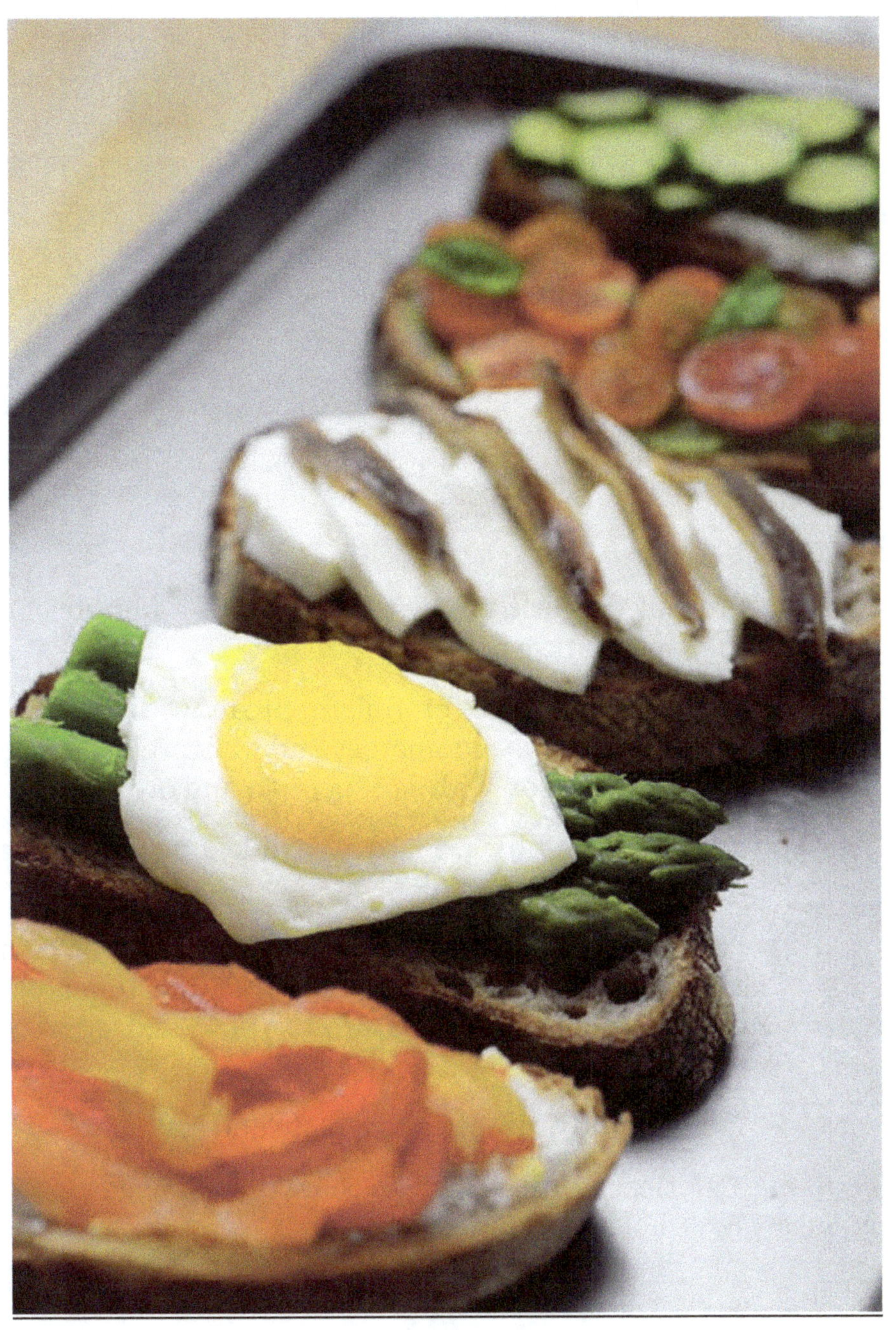

Preparation Time : 5 minutes

Cooking Time : 10 minutes

Servings : 2

Ingredients :

- 4 slices of Italian bread
- 1 cup chopped tomato tea
- 1 cup grated mozzarella tea
- Olive oil
- Oregano, salt, and pepper
- 4 fresh basil leaves

Directions :

1. Preheat the air fryer. Set the timer of 5 minutes and the temperature to 2000C.

2. Sprinkle the slices of Italian bread with olive oil. Divide the chopped tomatoes and mozzarella between the slices. Season with salt, pepper, and oregano.

3. Put oil in the filling. Place a basil leaf on top of each slice.

4. Put the bruschetta in the basket of the air fryer being careful not to spill the filling. Set the timer of 5 minutes, set the temperature to 180C, and press the power button.

5. Transfer the bruschetta to a plate and serve.

Nutrition : Calories: 434; Fat: 14g; Carbohydrates: 63g; Protein: 11g; Sugar: 8g; Cholesterol: 0mg

Cream Buns with Strawberries

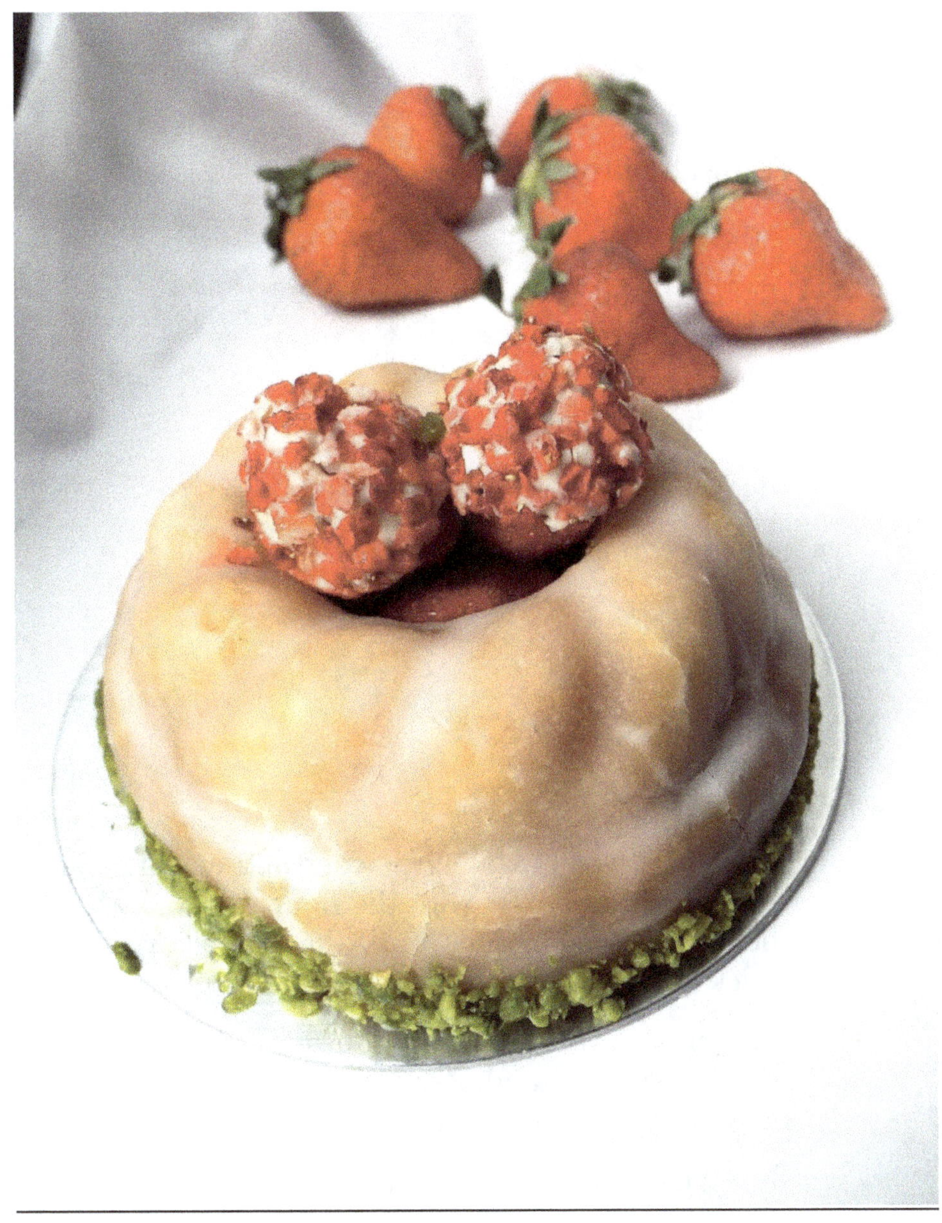

<u>*Preparation Time*</u> : 10 minutes

<u>*Cooking Time*</u> : 12 minutes

<u>*Servings*</u> : 6

<u>*Ingredients*</u> :

- 240g all-purpose flour
- 50g granulated sugar
- 8g baking powder
- 1g of salt
- 85g chopped cold butter
- 84g chopped fresh strawberries
- 120 ml whipping cream
- 2 large eggs
- 10 ml vanilla extract
- 5 ml of water

<u>*Directions*</u> :

1. Sift flour, sugar, baking powder and salt in a large bowl. Put the butter with the flour with the use of a blender or your hands until the mixture resembles thick crumbs.

2. Mix the strawberries in the flour mixture. Set aside for the mixture to stand. Beat the whipping cream, 1 egg and the vanilla extract in a separate bowl.

3. Put the cream mixture in the flour mixture until they are homogeneous, and then spread the mixture to a thickness of 38 mm.

4. Use a round cookie cutter to cut the buns. Spread the buns with a combination of egg and water. Set aside

5. Preheat the air fryer, set it to 180C.

6. Place baking paper in the preheated inner basket.

7. Place the buns on top of the baking paper and cook for 12 minutes at 180C, until golden brown.

Nutrition : Calories: 150; Fat: 14g; Carbohydrates: 3g; Protein: 11g; Sugar: 8g; Cholesterol: 0mg

Blueberry Buns

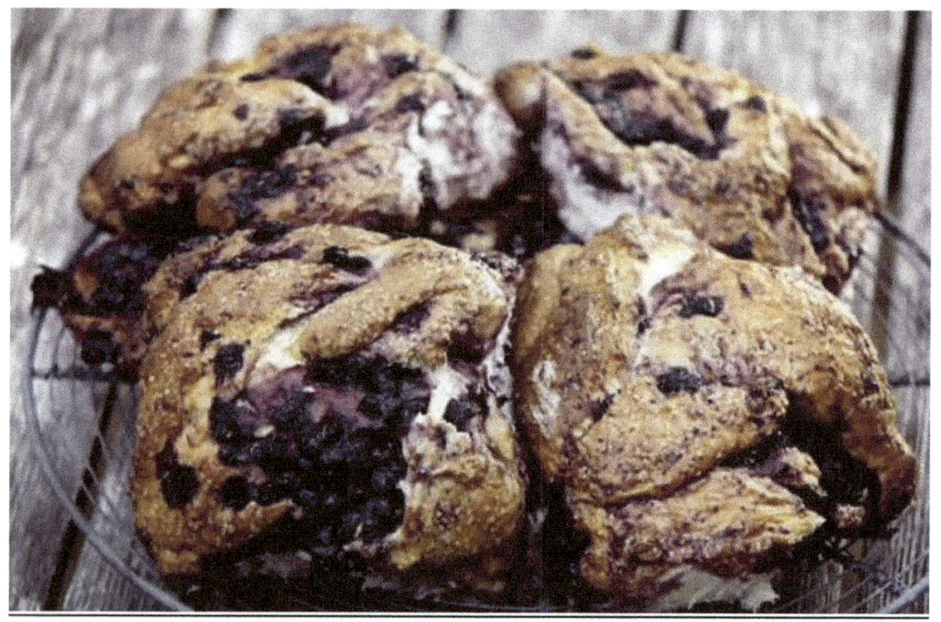

Preparation Time : 10 minutes

Cooking Time : 12 minutes

Servings : 6

Ingredients :

- 240g all-purpose flour
- 50g granulated sugar
- 8g baking powder
- 2g of salt
- 85g chopped cold butter
- 85g of fresh blueberries
- 3g grated fresh ginger
- 113 ml whipping cream
- 2 large eggs
- 4 ml vanilla extract
- 5 ml of water

Directions :

1. Put sugar, flour, baking powder and salt in a large bowl.

2. Put the butter with the flour using a blender or your hands until the mixture resembles thick crumbs.

3. Mix the blueberries and ginger in the flour mixture and set aside

4. Mix the whipping cream, 1 egg and the vanilla extract in a different container.

5. Put the cream mixture with the flour mixture until combined.

6. Shape the dough until it reaches a thickness of approximately 38 mm and cut it into eighths.

7. Spread the buns with a combination of egg and water. Set aside Preheat the air fryer set it to 180C.

8. Place baking paper in the preheated inner basket and place the buns on top of the paper. Cook for 12 minutes at 180C, until golden brown

Nutrition : Calories: 105; Fat: 1.64g; Carbohydrates: 20.09g; Protein: 2.43g; Sugar: 2.1g; Cholesterol: 0mg

Cauliflower Potato Mash

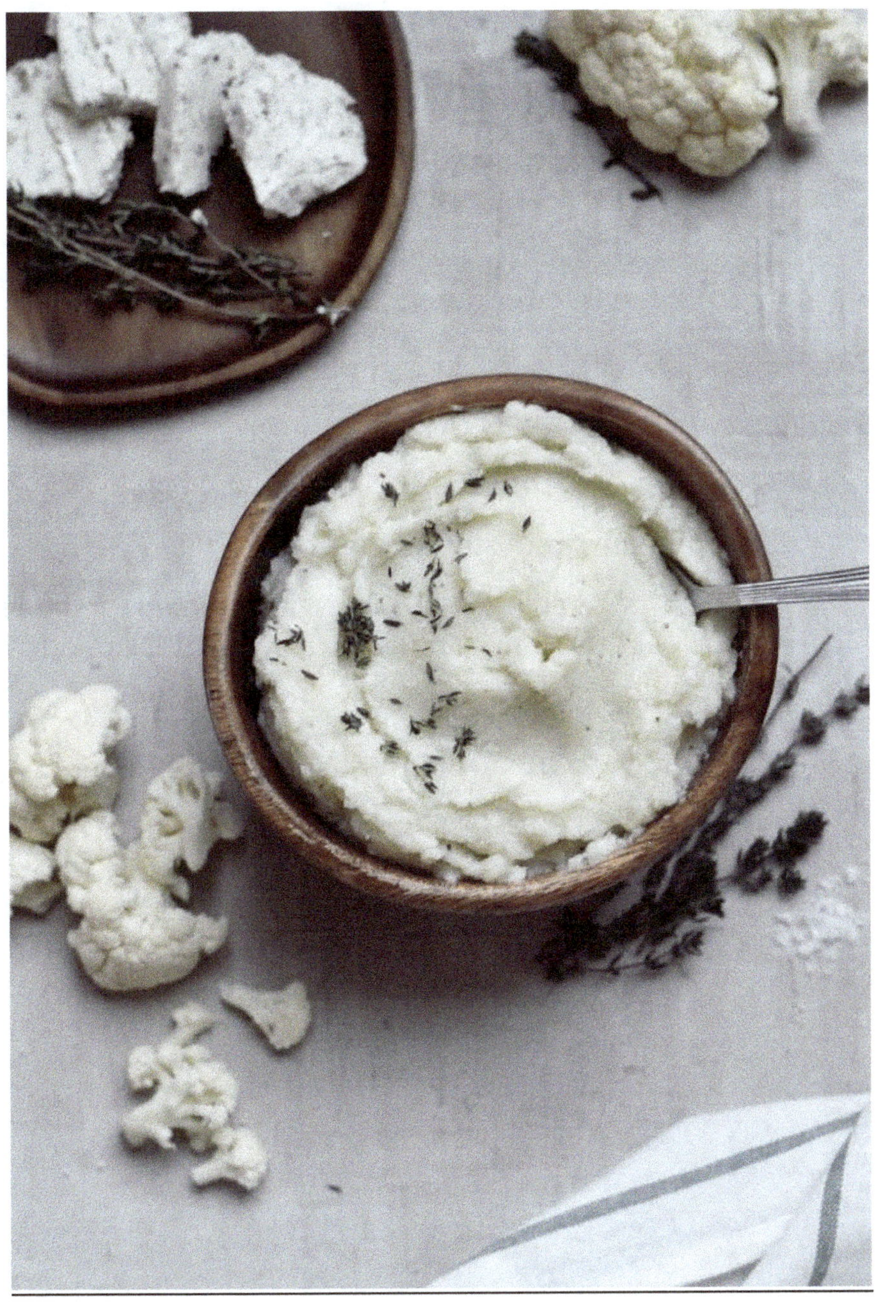

Preparation Time : 30 minutes Servings: 4

Cooking Time : 5 minutes

Ingredients :

- 2 cups potatoes, peeled and cubed
- 2 tbsp. butter
- ¼ cup milk
- 10 oz. cauliflower florets
- ¾ tsp. salt

Directions :

1. Add water to the saucepan and bring to boil.
2. Reduce heat and simmer for 10 minutes.
3. Drain vegetables well. Transfer vegetables, butter, milk, and salt in a blender and blend until smooth.
4. Serve and enjoy.

Nutrition : Calories 128; Fat 6.2 g; Sugar 3.3 g; Protein 3.2 g; Cholesterol 17 mg

French toast in Sticks

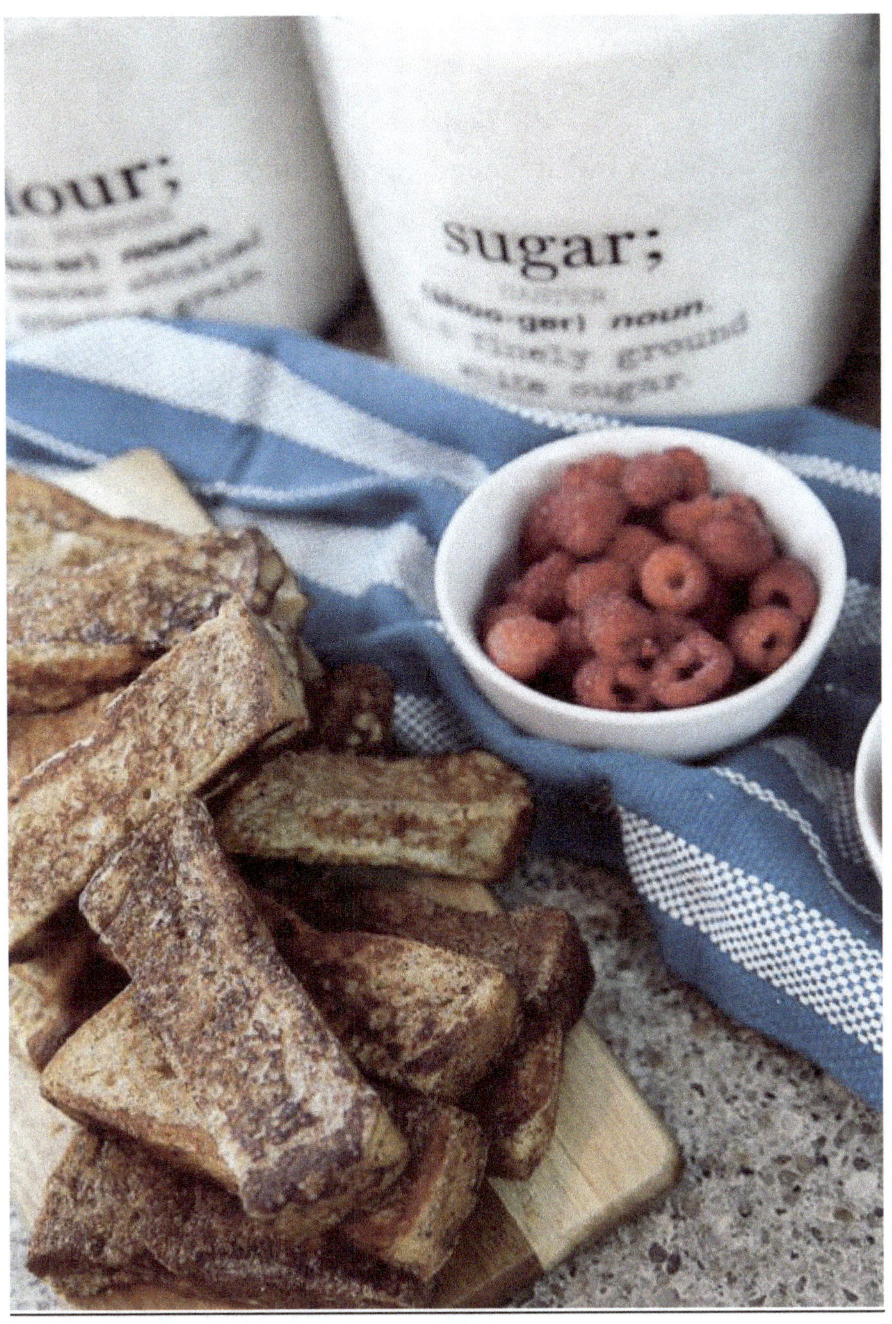

<u>*Preparation Time*</u> : 5 minutes

<u>*Cooking Time*</u> : 10 minutes

<u>*Servings*</u> : 4

<u>*Ingredients*</u> :

- 4 slices of white bread, 38 mm thick, preferably hard
- 2 eggs
- 60 ml of milk
- 15 ml maple sauce
- 2 ml vanilla extract
- Nonstick Spray Oil
- 38g of sugar
- 3ground cinnamon
- Maple syrup, to serve
- Sugar to sprinkle

<u>*Directions*</u> :

1. Cut each slice of bread into thirds making 12 pieces. Place sideways
2. Beat the eggs, milk, maple syrup and vanilla.
3. Preheat the air fryer, set it to 175C.
4. Dip the sliced bread in the egg mixture and place it in the preheated air fryer. Sprinkle French toast generously with oil spray.
5. Cook French toast for 10 minutes at 175C. Turn the toast halfway through cooking.

6. Mix the sugar and cinnamon in a bowl.

7. Cover the French toast with the sugar and cinnamon
    mixture when you have finished cooking.

8. Serve with Maple syrup and sprinkle with powdered
    sugar

Nutrition : Calories 128; Fat 6.2 g; Carbohydrates 16.3 g; Sugar
3.3 g; Protein 3.2 g; Cholesterol 17 mg

Muffins Sandwich

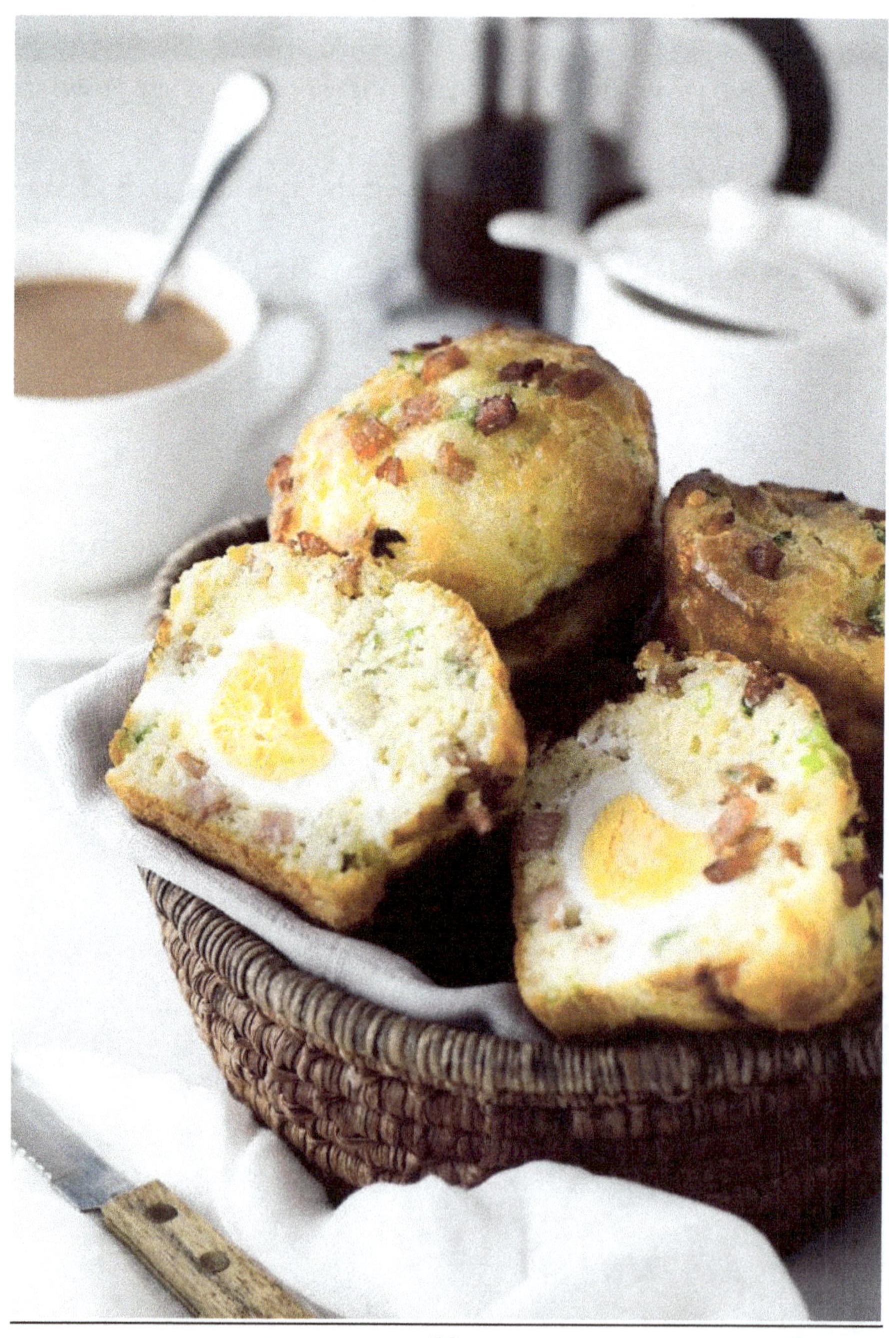

Preparation Time : 2 minutes

Cooking Time : 10 minutes

Servings : 1

Ingredients :

- Nonstick Spray Oil
- 1 slice of white cheddar cheese
- 1 slice of Canadian bacon
- 1 English muffin, divided
- 15 ml hot water
- 1 large egg
- Salt and pepper to taste

Directions :

1. Spray the inside of an 85g mold with oil spray and place it in the air fryer.
2. Preheat the air fryer, set it to 160C.
3. Add the Canadian cheese and bacon in the preheated air fryer.
4. Pour the hot water and the egg into the hot pan and season with salt and pepper.
5. Select Bread, set to 10 minutes.
6. Take out the English muffins after 7 minutes, leaving the egg for the full time.
7. Build your sandwich by placing the cooked egg on top of the English muffing and serve

<u>*Nutrition*</u> : Calories 400; Fat 26g; Carbohydrates 26g; Sugar 15 g; Protein 3 g; Cholesterol 155 mg

Bacon BBQ

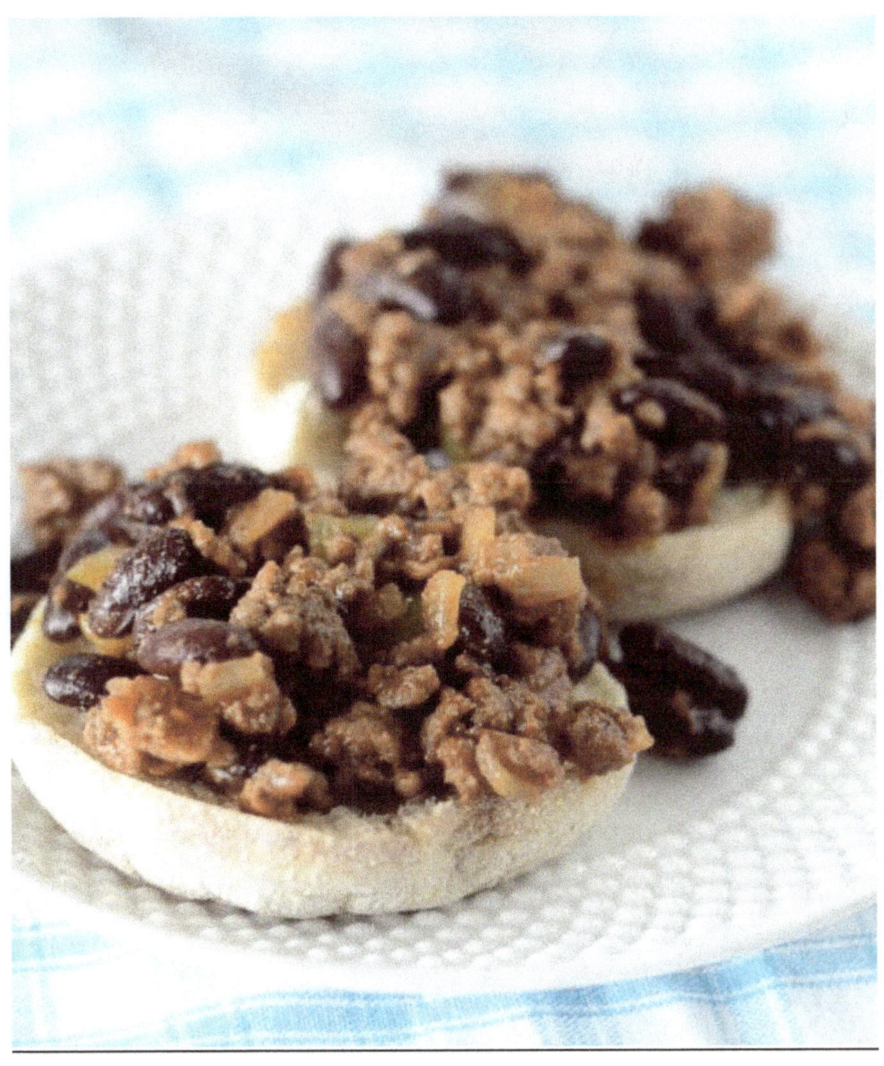

Preparation Time : 2 minutes

Cooking Time : 8 minutes

Servings : 2

Ingredients :

- 13g dark brown sugar
- 5g chili powder
- 1g ground cumin
- 1g cayenne pepper
- 4 slices of bacon, cut in half

Directions :

1. Mix seasonings until well combined.
2. Dip the bacon in the dressing until it is completely covered. Leave aside.
3. Preheat the air fryer, set it to 160C.
4. Place the bacon in the preheated air fryer
5. Select Bacon and press Start/Pause.

Nutrition : Calories: 1124; Fat: 72g; Carbohydrates: 59g; Protein: 49g; Sugar: 11g; Cholesterol: 77mg

Stuffed French toast

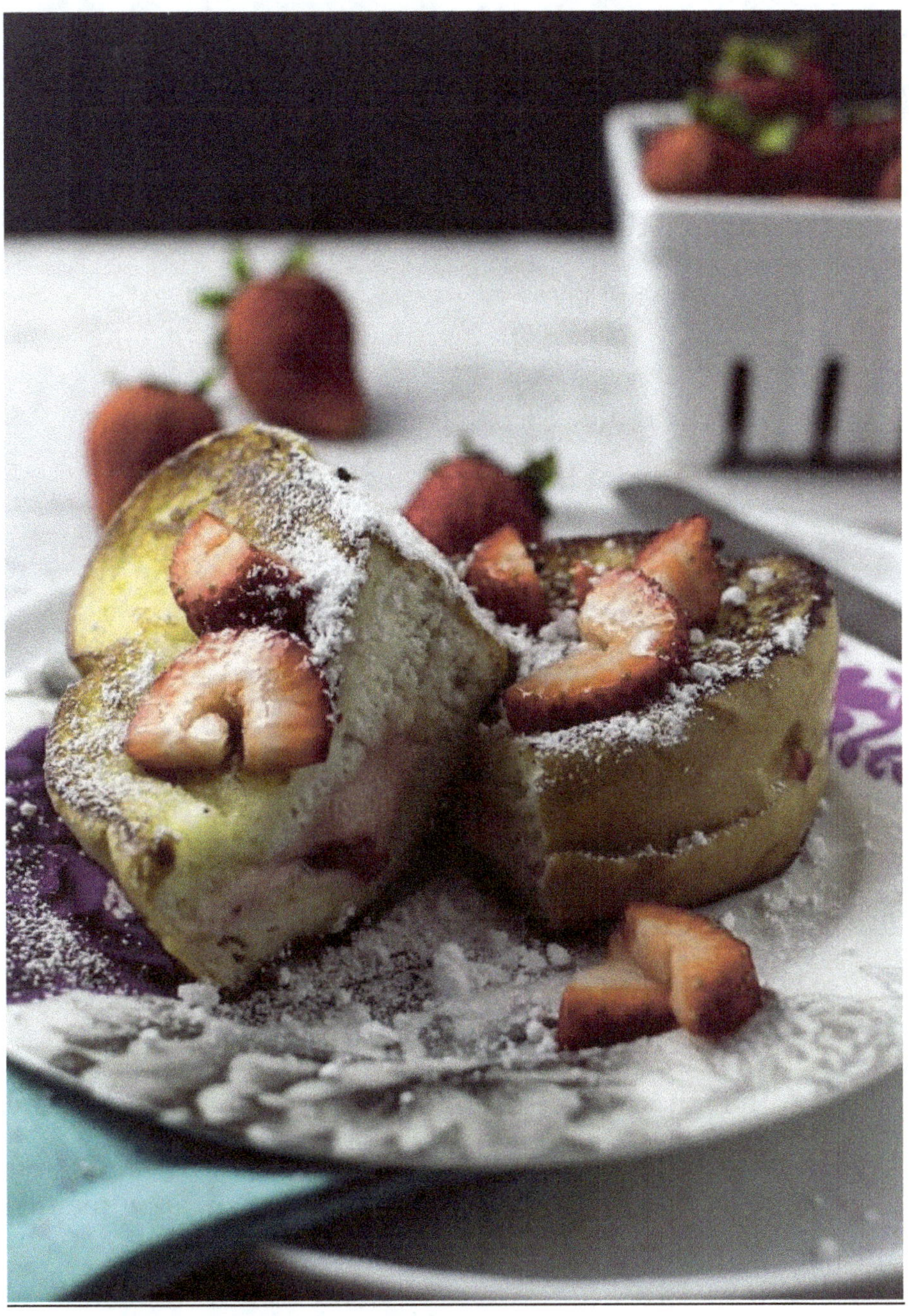

Preparation Time : 4 minutes

Cooking Time : 10 minutes

Servings : 1

Ingredients :

- 1 slice of brioche bread,
- 64 mm thick, preferably rancid
- 113g cream cheese
- 2 eggs
- 15 ml of milk
- 30 ml whipping cream
- 38g of sugar
- 3g cinnamon
- 2 ml vanilla extract
- Nonstick Spray Oil
- Pistachios chopped to cover
- Maple syrup, to serve

Directions :

1. Preheat the air fryer, set it to 175C.
2. Cut a slit in the middle of the muffin.
3. Fill the inside of the slit with cream cheese. Leave aside.
4. Mix the eggs, milk, whipping cream, sugar, cinnamon, and vanilla extract.

5. Moisten the stuffed French toast in the egg mixture for 10 seconds on each side.

6. Sprinkle each side of French toast with oil spray.

7. Place the French toast in the preheated air fryer and cook for 10 minutes at 175C

8. Stir the French toast carefully with a spatula when you finish cooking.

9. Serve topped with chopped pistachios and acrid syrup.

Nutrition : Calories: 159; Fat: 7.5g; Carbohydrates: 25.2g; Protein: 14g; Sugar: 0g; Cholesterol: 90mg

Chili Chicken Wings

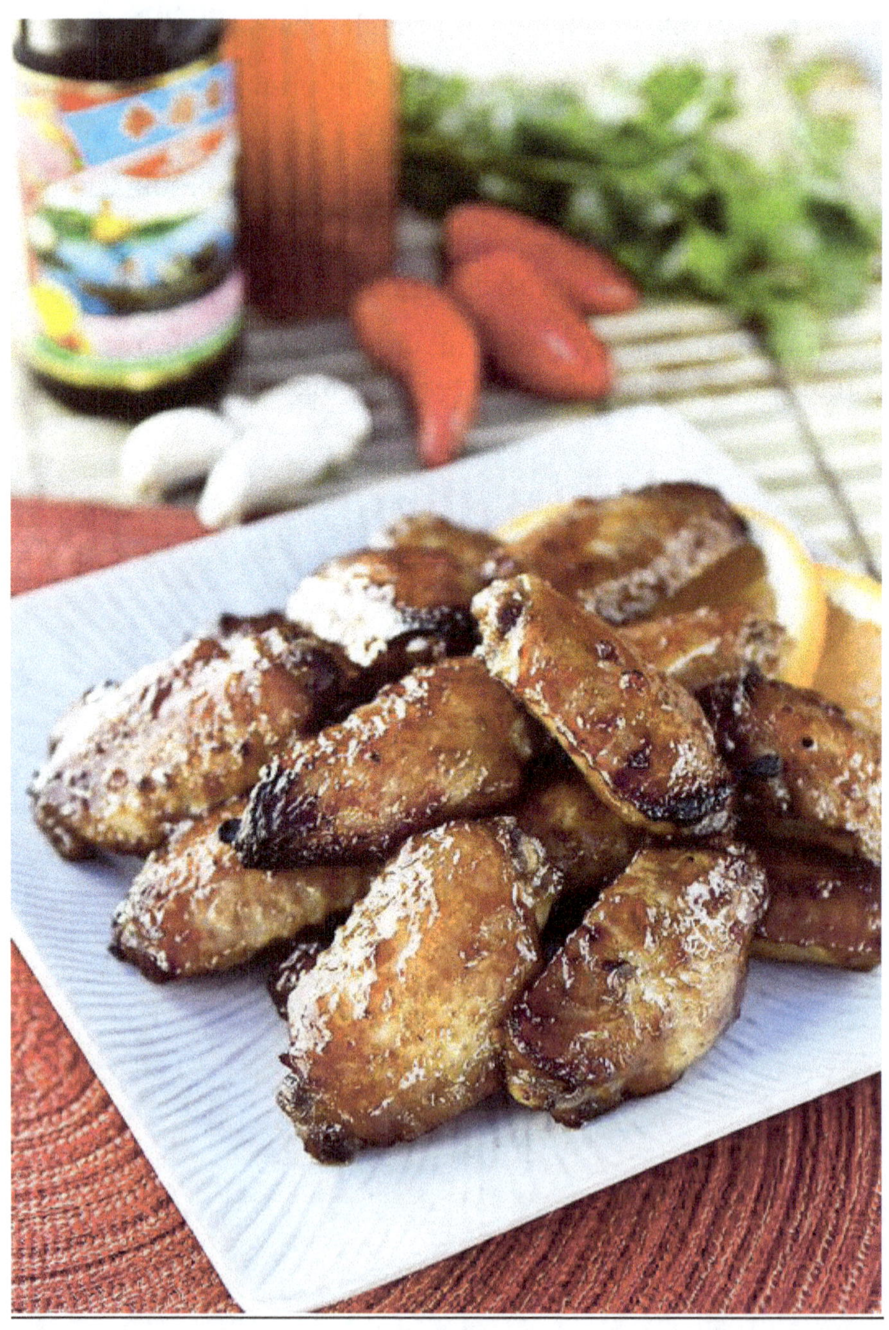

Preparation Time : 10 minutes

Cooking Time : 1 hour 10 minutes

Servings : 4

Ingredients :

- 2 lbs. chicken wings
- 1/8 tsp. paprika
- 1/2 cup coconut flour
- 1/4 tsp. garlic powder
- 1/4 tsp. chili powder

Directions :

1. Preheat the oven to 400 F/ 200 C.
2. In a mixing bowl, add all ingredients except chicken wings and mix well.
3. Add chicken wings to the bowl mixture and coat well and place on a baking tray.
4. Bake in preheated oven for 55-60 minutes.
5. Serve and enjoy.

Nutrition : Calories 440; Fat 17.1 g; Carbohydrates 1.3 g; Sugar 0.2 g; Protein 65.9 g; Cholesterol 202 mg

Garlic Chicken Wings

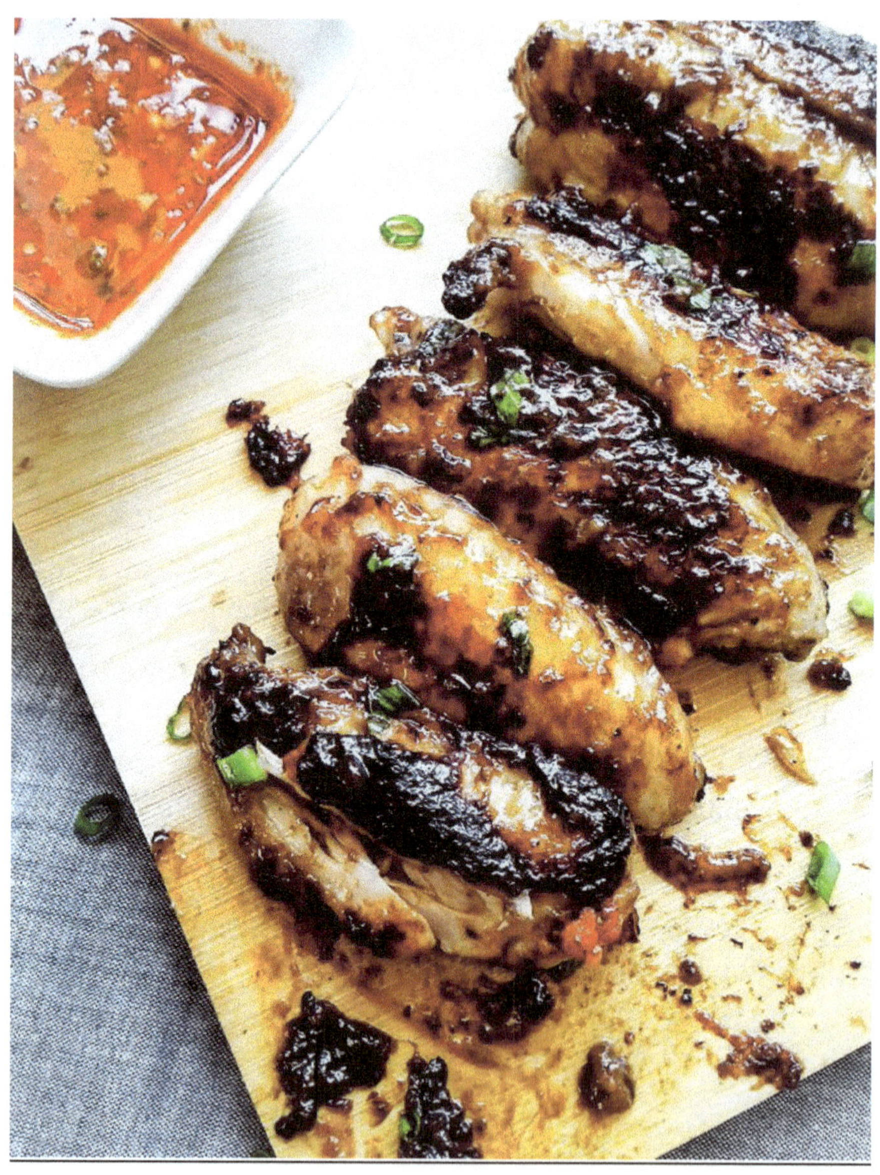

<u>*Preparation Time*</u> : 10 minutes

<u>*Cooking Time*</u> : 55 minutes

<u>*Servings*</u> : 6

<u>*Ingredients*</u> :

- 12 chicken wings
- 2 garlic cloves, minced
- 3 tbsp. ghee
- 1/2 tsp. turmeric
- 2 tsp. cumin seeds

<u>*Directions*</u> :

1. Preheat the oven to 425 F/ 215 C.
2. In a large bowl, mix together 1 teaspoon cumin, 1 tbsp. ghee, turmeric, pepper, and salt.
3. Add chicken wings to the bowl and toss well.
4. Spread chicken wings on a baking tray and bake in preheated oven for 30 minutes.
5. Turn chicken wings to another side and bake for 8 minutes more.
6. Meanwhile, heat remaining ghee in a pan over medium heat.
7. Add garlic and cumin to the pan and cook for a minute.
8. Remove pan from heat and set aside.
9. Remove chicken wings from oven and drizzle with ghee mixture
10. Bake chicken wings 5 minutes more.

11. Serve and enjoy.

Nutrition : Calories 378; Fat 27.9 g; Carbohydrates 11.4 g; Sugar 0 g; Protein 19.7 g; Cholesterol 94 mg

Spinach Cheese Pie

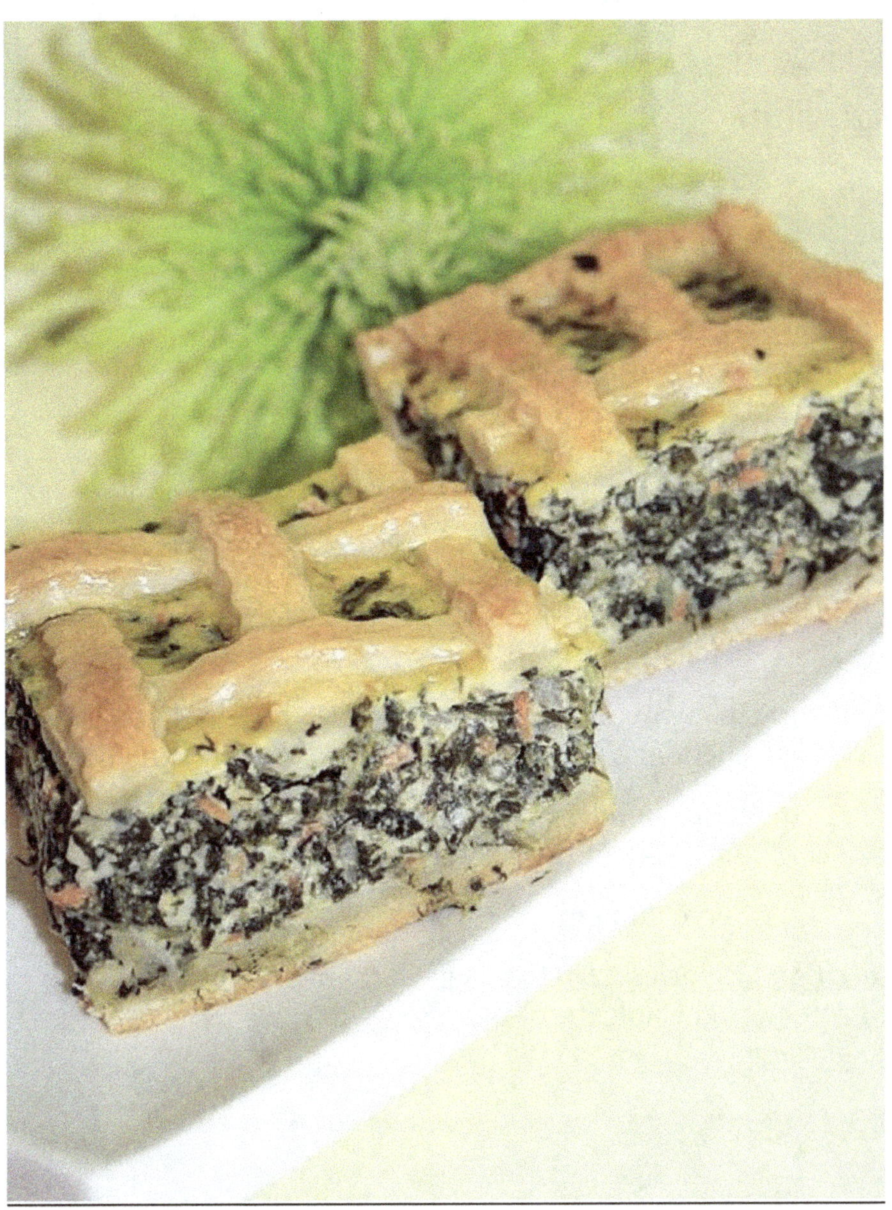

<u>Preparation Time</u> : 10 minutes

<u>Cooking Time</u> : 40 minutes

<u>Servings</u> : 8

<u>Ingredients</u> :

- 6 eggs, lightly beaten
- 2 boxes frozen spinach, chopped
- 2 cup cheddar cheese, shredded
- 15 oz. cottage cheese
- 1 tsp. salt

<u>Directions</u> :

1. Preheat the oven to 375 F/ 190 C.
2. Spray an 8*8-inch baking dish with cooking spray and set aside.
3. In a mixing bowl, combine together spinach, eggs, cheddar cheese, cottage cheese, pepper, and salt.
4. Pour spinach mixture into the prepared baking dish and bake in preheated oven for 10 minutes.
5. Serve and enjoy.

<u>Nutrition</u> : Calories 229; Fat 14 g; Carbohydrates 5.4 g; Sugar 0.9 g; Protein 21 g; Cholesterol 157 mg

Tasty Harissa Chicken

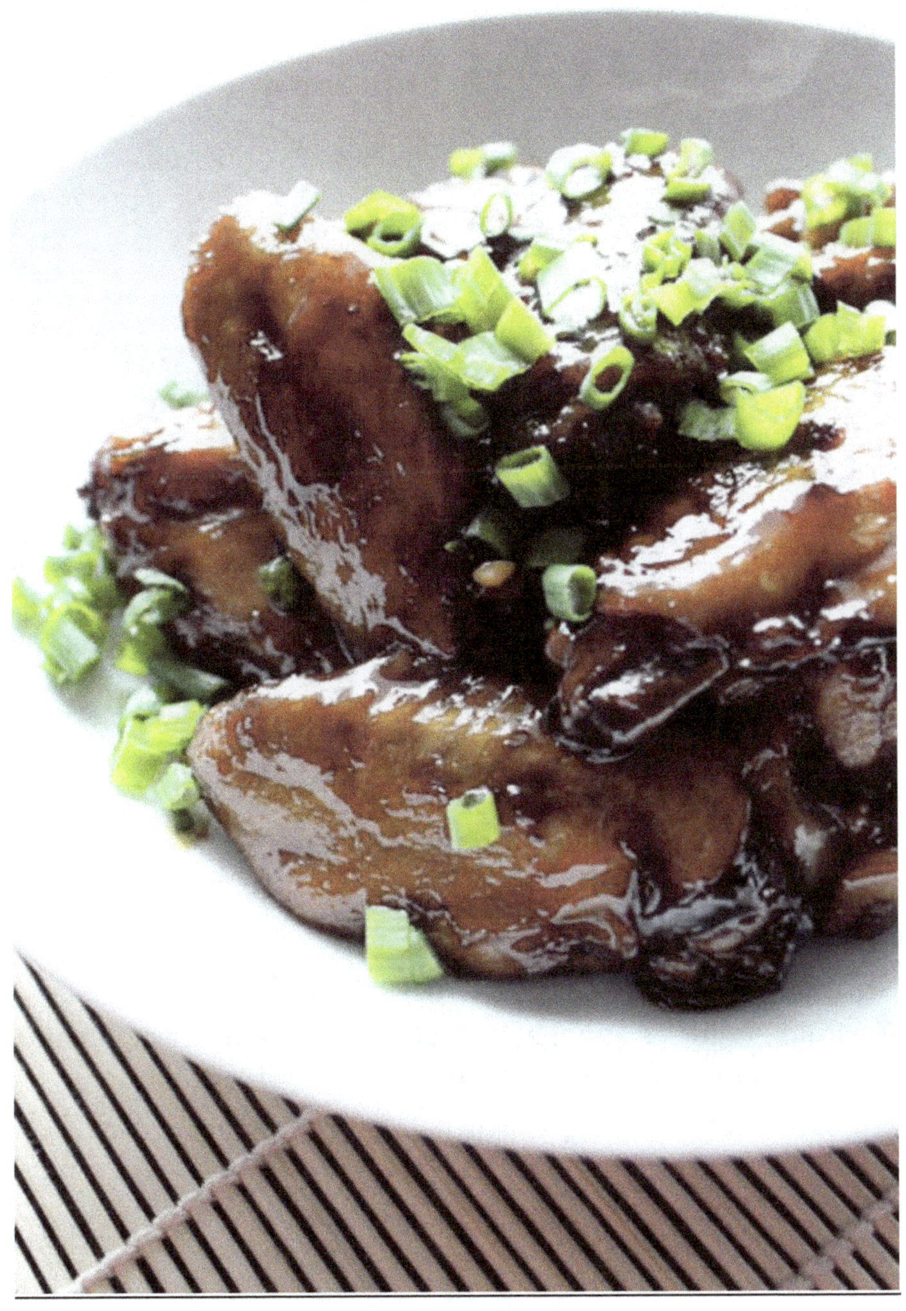

Preparation Time : 10 minutes

Cooking Time : 4 hours 10 minutes

Servings : 4

Ingredients :

- 1 lb. chicken breasts, skinless and boneless
- 1/2 tsp. ground cumin
- 1 cup harissa sauce
- 1/4 tsp. garlic powder
- 1/2 tsp. kosher salt

Directions :

1. Season chicken with garlic powder, cumin, and salt.
2. Place chicken to the slow cooker.
3. Pour harissa sauce over the chicken.
4. Cover slow cooker with lid and cook on low for 4 hours.
5. Remove chicken from slow cooker and shred using a fork.
6. Return shredded chicken to the slow cooker and stir well.
7. Serve and enjoy.

Nutrition : Calories 232; Fat 9.7 g; Carbohydrates 1.3 g; Sugar 0.1 g; Protein 32.9 g; Cholesterol 101 mg

Roasted Balsamic Mushrooms

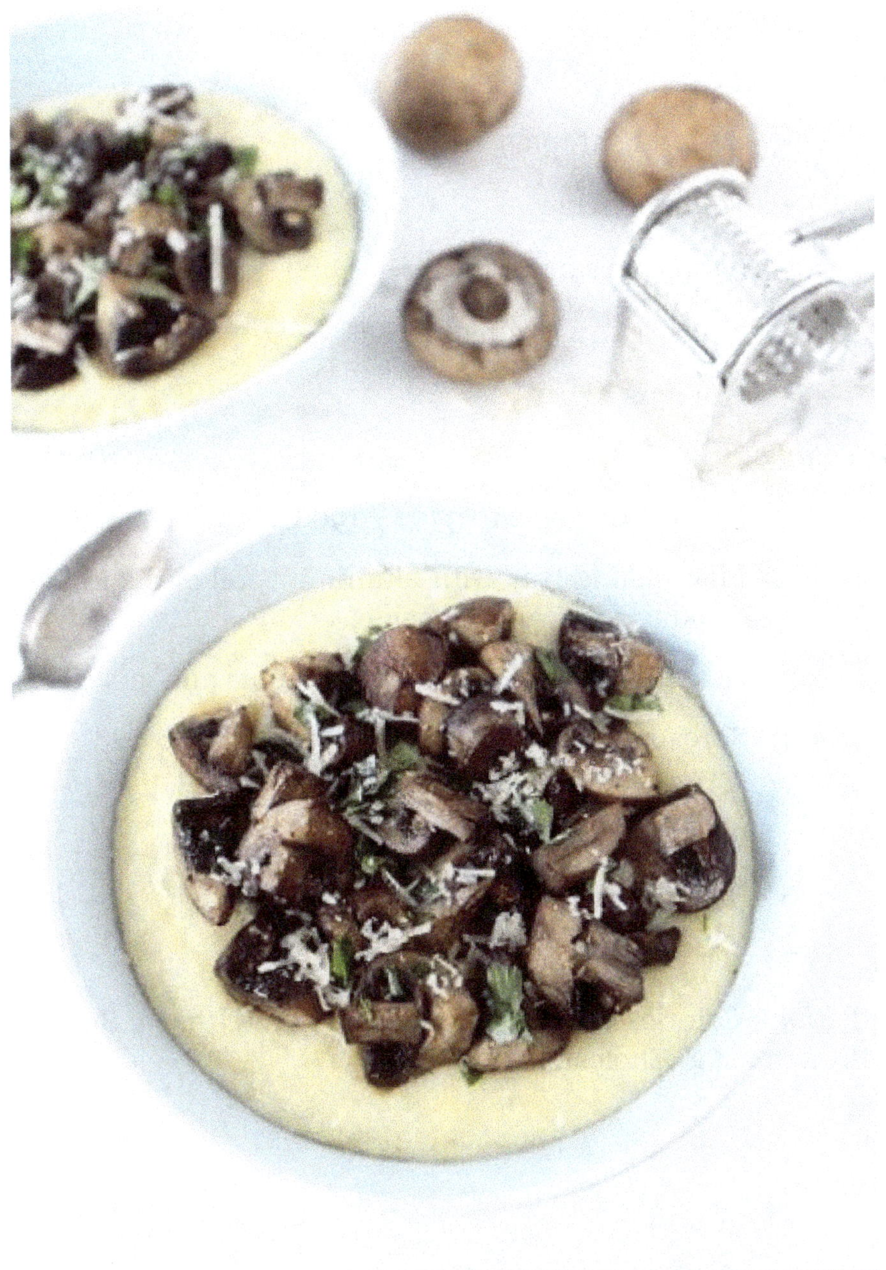

Preparation Time : 10 minutes

Cooking Time : 50 minutes

Servings : 4

Ingredients :

- 8 oz. mushrooms, sliced
- 1/2 tsp. thyme
- 2 tbsp. balsamic vinegar
- 2 tbsp. extra virgin olive oil
- 2 onions, sliced

Directions :

1. Preheat the oven to 375 F/ 190 C.
2. Line baking tray with aluminum foil and spray with cooking spray and set aside.
3. In a mixing bowl, add all ingredients and mix well.
4. Spread mushroom mixture onto a prepared baking tray.
5. Roast in preheated oven for 45 minutes.
6. Season with pepper and salt.
7. Serve and enjoy.

Nutrition : Calories 96; Fat 7.2 g; Carbohydrates 7.2 g; Sugar 3.3 g; Protein 2.4 g; Cholesterol 0 mg

Chia Crackers

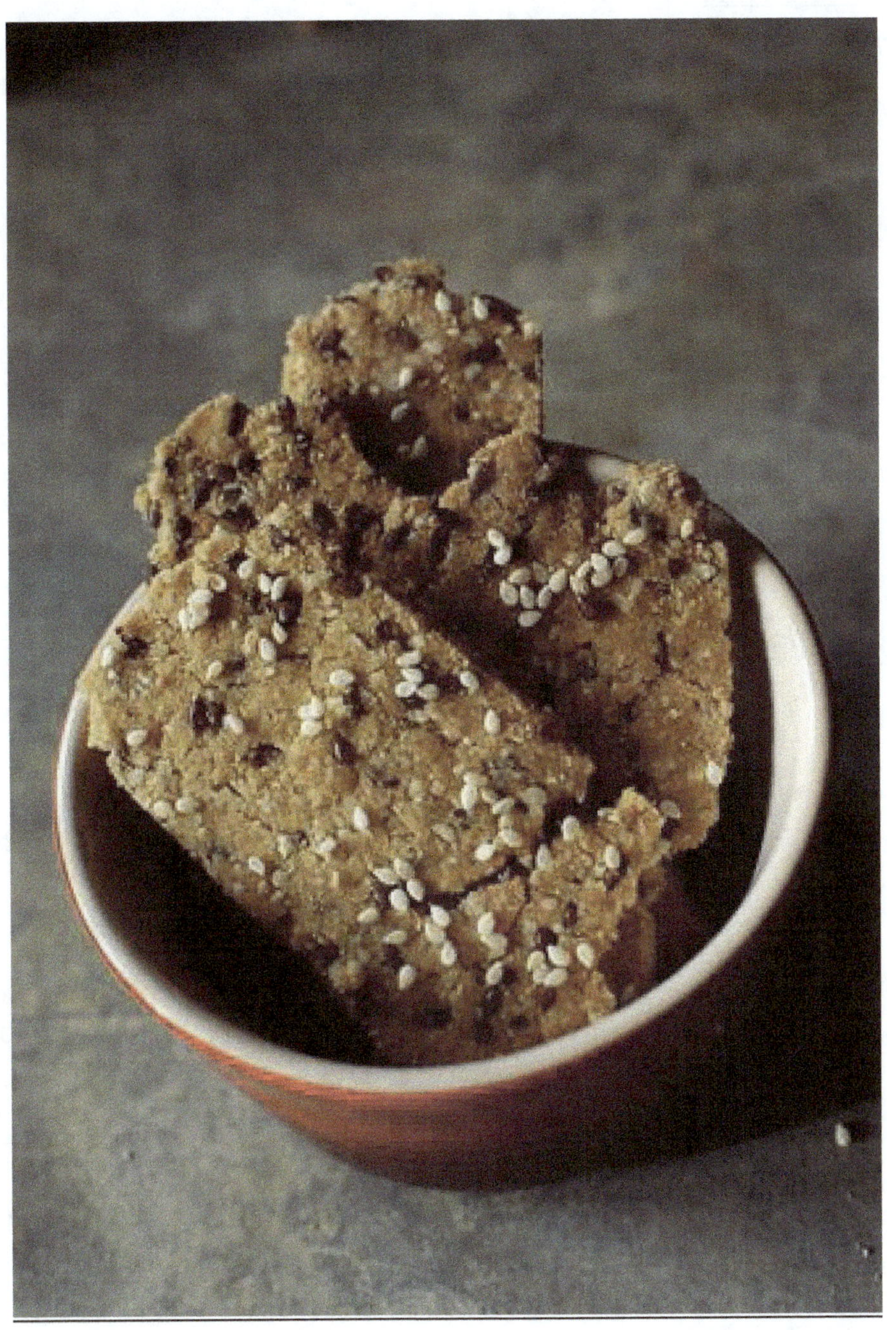

Preparation Time : 20 minutes

Cooking Time : 1 hour

Servings : 24-26 crackers

Ingredients :

- 1/2 cup pecans, chopped
- 1/2 cup chia seeds
- 1/2 teaspoon cayenne pepper
- 1 cup water
- 1/4 cup Nutritional yeast
- 1/2 cup pumpkin seeds
- 1/4 cup ground flax
- Salt and pepper, to taste

Directions :

1. Mix around 1/2 cup chia seeds and 1 cup water. Keep it aside.

2. Take another bowl and combine all the remaining Ingredients. Combine well and stir in the chia water mixture until you obtained dough.

3. Transfer the dough onto a baking sheet and rollout (¼" thick).

4. Transfer into a preheated oven at 325°F and bake for about half an hour.

5. Take out from the oven, flip over the dough, and cut it into desired cracker shape/squares.

6. Spread and back again for further half an hour, or until crispy and browned.

7. Once done, take out from oven and let them cool at room temperature. Enjoy!

<u>*Nutrition*</u> : 41 calories; 3.1g Fat; 2g Total Carbohydrates; 2g Protein

Orange- Spiced Pumpkin Hummus

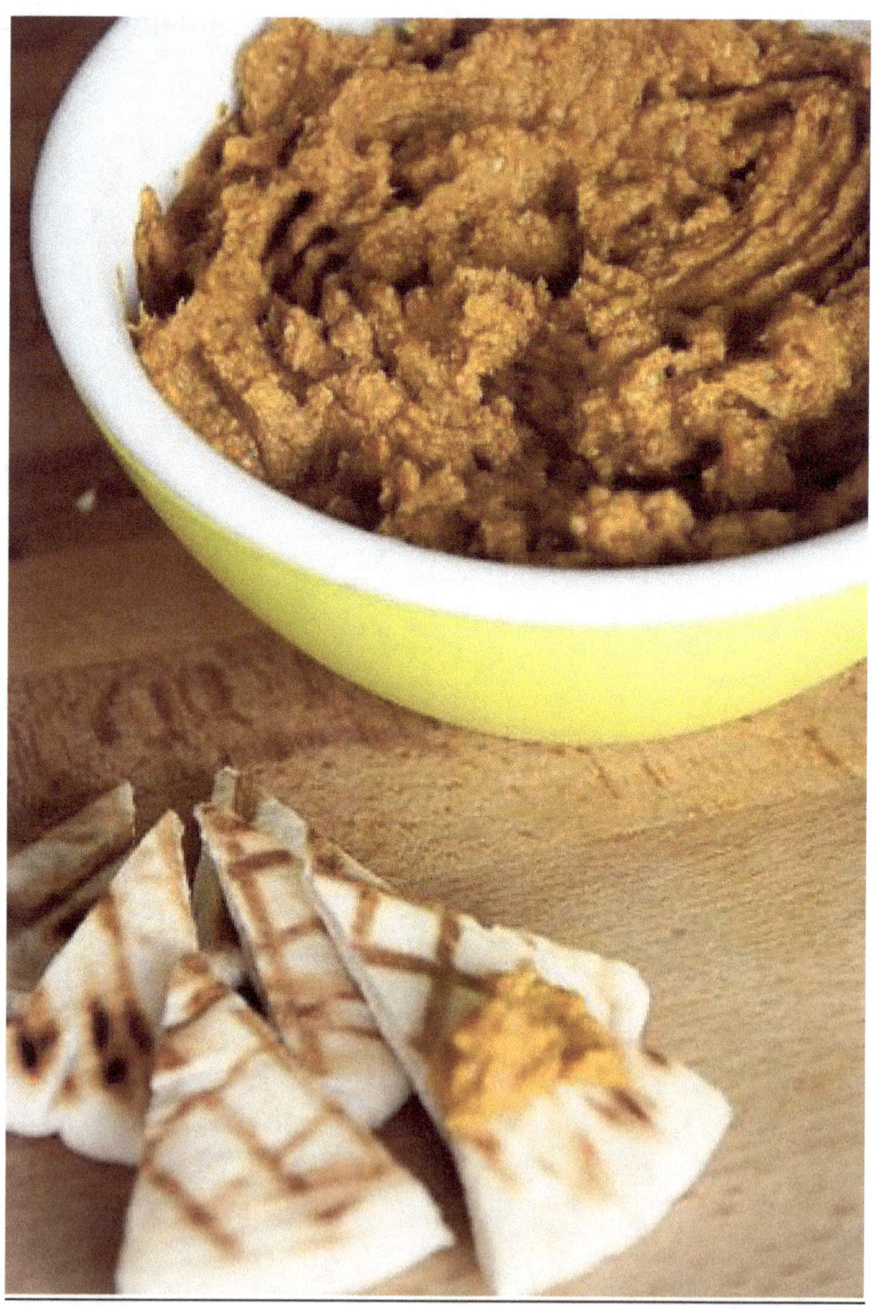

Preparation Time : 2 minutes

Cooking Time : 5 minutes

Servings : 4 cups

Ingredients :

- 1 tablespoon maple syrup
- 1/2 teaspoon salt
- 1 can (16oz.) garbanzo beans,
- 1/8 teaspoon ginger or nutmeg
- 1 cup canned pumpkin Blend,
- 1/8 teaspoon cinnamon
- 1/4 cup tahini
- 1 tablespoon fresh orange juice
- Pinch of orange zest, for garnish
- 1 tablespoon apple cider vinegar

Directions :

1. Mix all the Ingredients to a food processor blender and blend until slightly chunky.

2. Serve right away and enjoy!

Nutrition : 291 Calories; 22.9g Fat; 15g Total Carbohydrates; 12g Protein

Cinnamon Maple Sweet Potato Bites

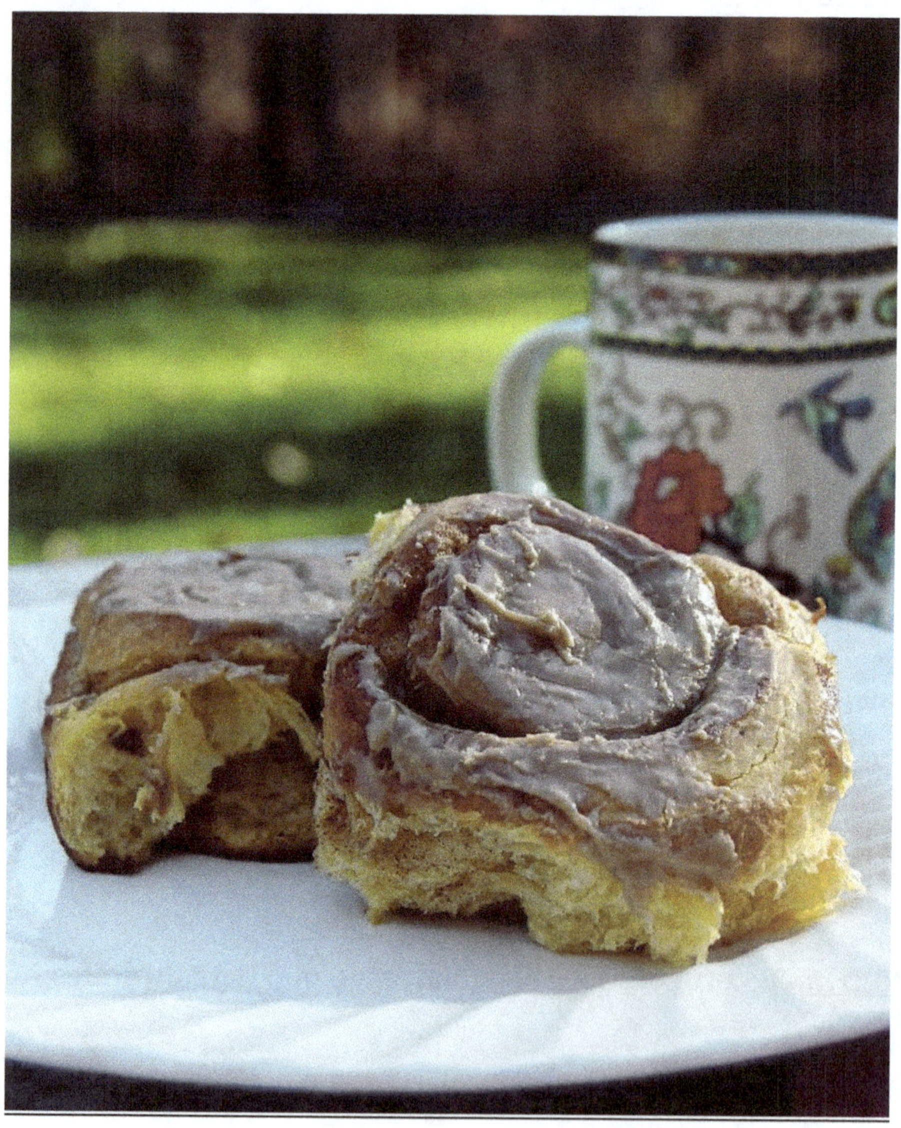

Preparation Time : 5 minutes

Cooking Time : 25 minutes

Servings : 3 to 4

Ingredients :

- ½ teaspoon corn-starch
- 1 teaspoon cinnamon
- 4 medium sweet potatoes, then peeled, and cut into bite-size cubes
- 2 to 3 tablespoons maple syrup
- 3 tablespoons butter, melted

Directions :

1. Transfer the potato cubes to a Ziploc bag and add in 3 tablespoons of melted butter. Seal and shake well until the potato cubes are coated with butter.

2. Add in the remaining Ingredients and shake again.

3. Transfer the potato cubes to a parchment-lined baking sheet. Cubes shouldn't be stacked on one another.

4. Sprinkle with cinnamon, if needed, and bake in a preheated oven at 425°F for about 25 to 30 minutes, stirring once during cooking.

5. Once done, take them out and stand at room temperature. Enjoy!

Nutrition : 436 Calories; 17.4g Fat; 71.8g Total Carbohydrates; 4.1g Protein

Cheesy Kale Chips

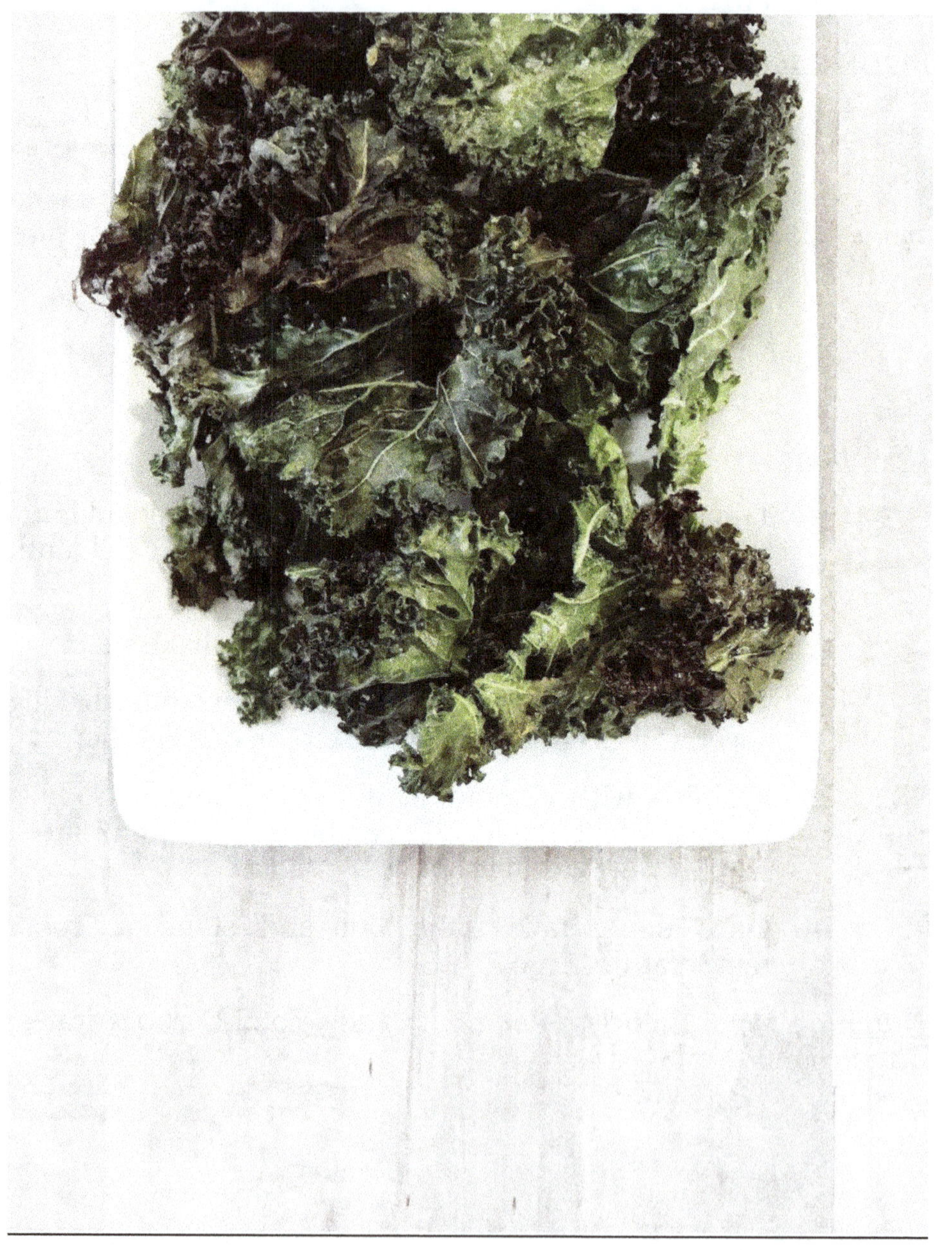

Preparation Time : 3 minutes

Cooking Time : 12 minutes

Servings : 4

Ingredients :

- 3 tablespoons Nutritional yeast
- 1 head curly kale, washed, ribs
- 3/4 teaspoon garlic powder
- 1 tablespoon olive oil
- 1 teaspoon onion powder
- Salt, to taste

Directions :

1. Line cookie sheets with parchment paper.
2. Drain the kale leaves and spread on a paper removed and leaves torn into chip-
3. towel. Then, kindly transfer the leaves to a bowl and sized pieces
4. add in 1 teaspoon onion powder, 3 tablespoons Nutritional yeast, 1 tablespoon olive oil, and 3/4
5. teaspoon garlic powder. Mix with your hands.
6. Spread the kale onto prepared cookie sheets. They shouldn't touch each other.
7. Bake into a preheated oven for about 350 F for about 10to 12 minutes.
8. Once crisp, take out from the oven, and sprinkle with a bit of salt. Serve and enjoy!

Nutrition : 71 Calories; 4g Fat; 5g Total Carbohydrates; 4g Protein

Lemon Roasted Bell Pepper

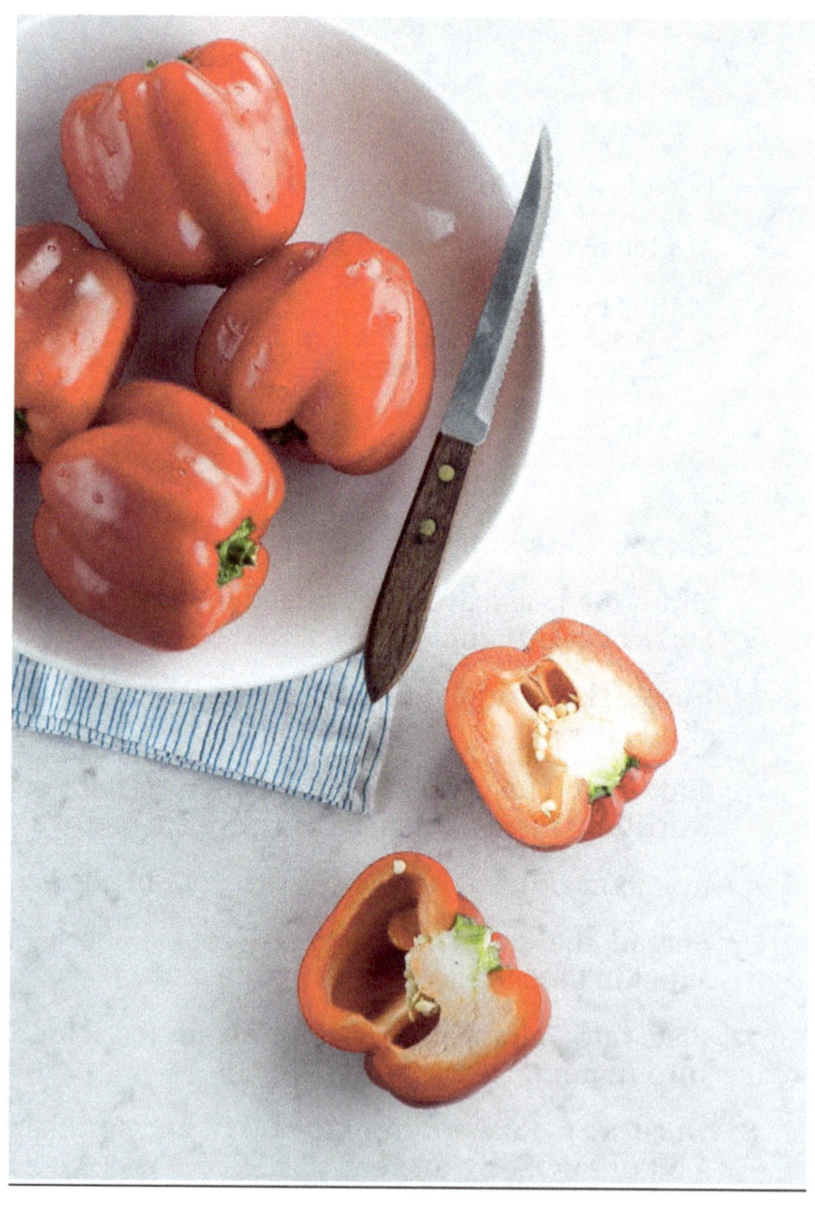

Preparation Time : 10 minutes

Cooking Time : 5 minutes

Servings : 4

Ingredients :

- 4 bell peppers
- 1 teaspoon olive oil
- 1 tablespoon mango juice
- 1/4 teaspoon garlic, minced
- 1 teaspoons oregano
- 1 pinch salt
- 1 pinch pepper

Directions :

1. Start heating the Air Fryer to 390 degrees F
2. Place some bell pepper in the Air fryer
3. Drizzle it with the olive oil and air fry for 5 minutes
4. Take a serving plate and transfer it
5. Take a small bowl and add garlic, oregano, mango juice, salt, and pepper
6. Mix them well and drizzle the mixture over the peppers
7. Serve and enjoy!

Nutrition : Calories: 59 kcal; Carbohydrates: 6 g; Fat: 5 g; Protein: 4 g

Subtle Roasted Mushrooms

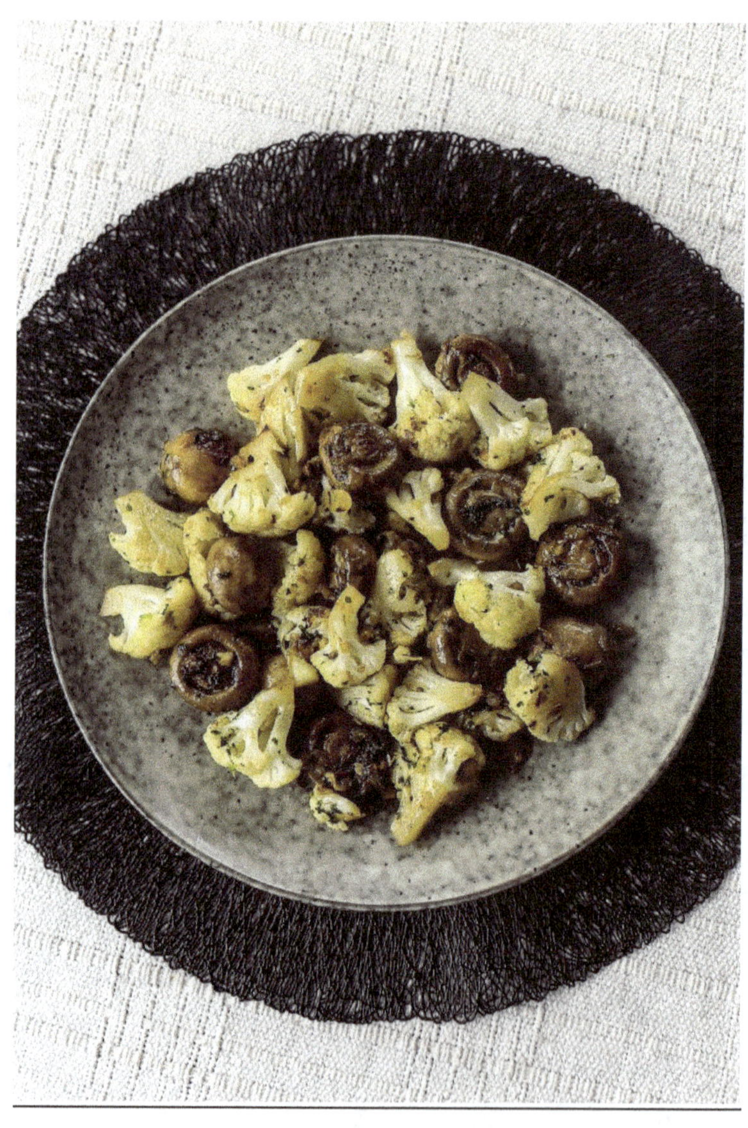

Preparation Time : 10 minutes

Cooking Time : 5 minutes

Servings :4

Ingredients :

- 2 teaspoons mixed Sebi Friendly herbs
- 1 tablespoon olive oil
- 1/2 teaspoon garlic powder
- 2 pounds mushrooms
- 2 tablespoons date sugar

Directions :

1. Wash mushrooms and turn dry in a plate of mixed greens spinner
2. Quarter them and put in a safe spot
3. Put garlic, oil, and spices in the dish of your oar type air fryer
4. Warmth for 2 minutes
5. Stir it.
6. Add some mushrooms and cook 25 minutes
7. Then include vermouth and cook for 5 minutes more
8. Serve and enjoy!

Nutrition : Calories: 94 kcal; Carbohydrates: 3 g; Fat: 8 g; Protein: 2 g

Fancy Spelt Bread

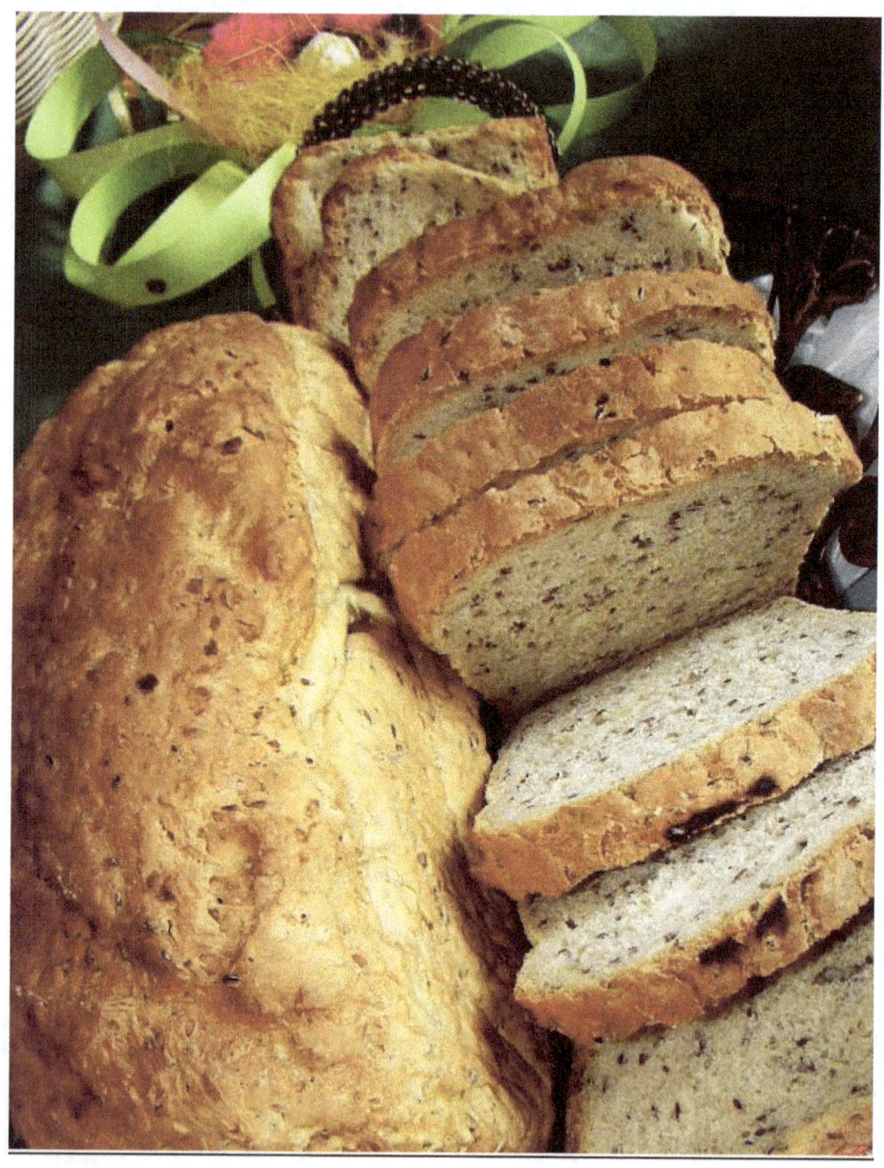

<u>*Preparation Time*</u> : 10 minutes

<u>*Cooking Time*</u> : 5 minutes

<u>*Servings*</u> :4

<u>*Ingredients*</u> :

- 1 cup spring water
- 1/2 cup of coconut milk
- 3 tablespoons avocado oil
- 1 teaspoon baking soda
- 1 tablespoon agave nectar
- 4 and 1/2 cups spelt flour
- 1 and 1/2 teaspoon salt

<u>*Directions*</u> :

1. Pre-heat your Air Fryer to 355 degrees F
2. Take a big bowl and add baking soda, salt, flour whisk well
3. Add 3/4 cup of water, plus coconut milk, oil and mix well
4. Sprinkle your working surface with flour, add dough to the flour
5. Roll well
6. Knead for about three minutes, adding small amounts of flour until dough is a nice ball
7. Place parchment paper in your cooking basket
8. Lightly grease your pan and put the dough inside
9. Transfer into Air Fryer and bake for 30-45 minutes until done

10. Remove then insert a stick to check for doneness

11. If done already serve and enjoy, if not, let it cook for a few minutes more

Nutrition : Calories: 203 kcal; Carbohydrates: 37 g; Fat: 4g; Protein: 7 g

Crispy Crunchy Hummus

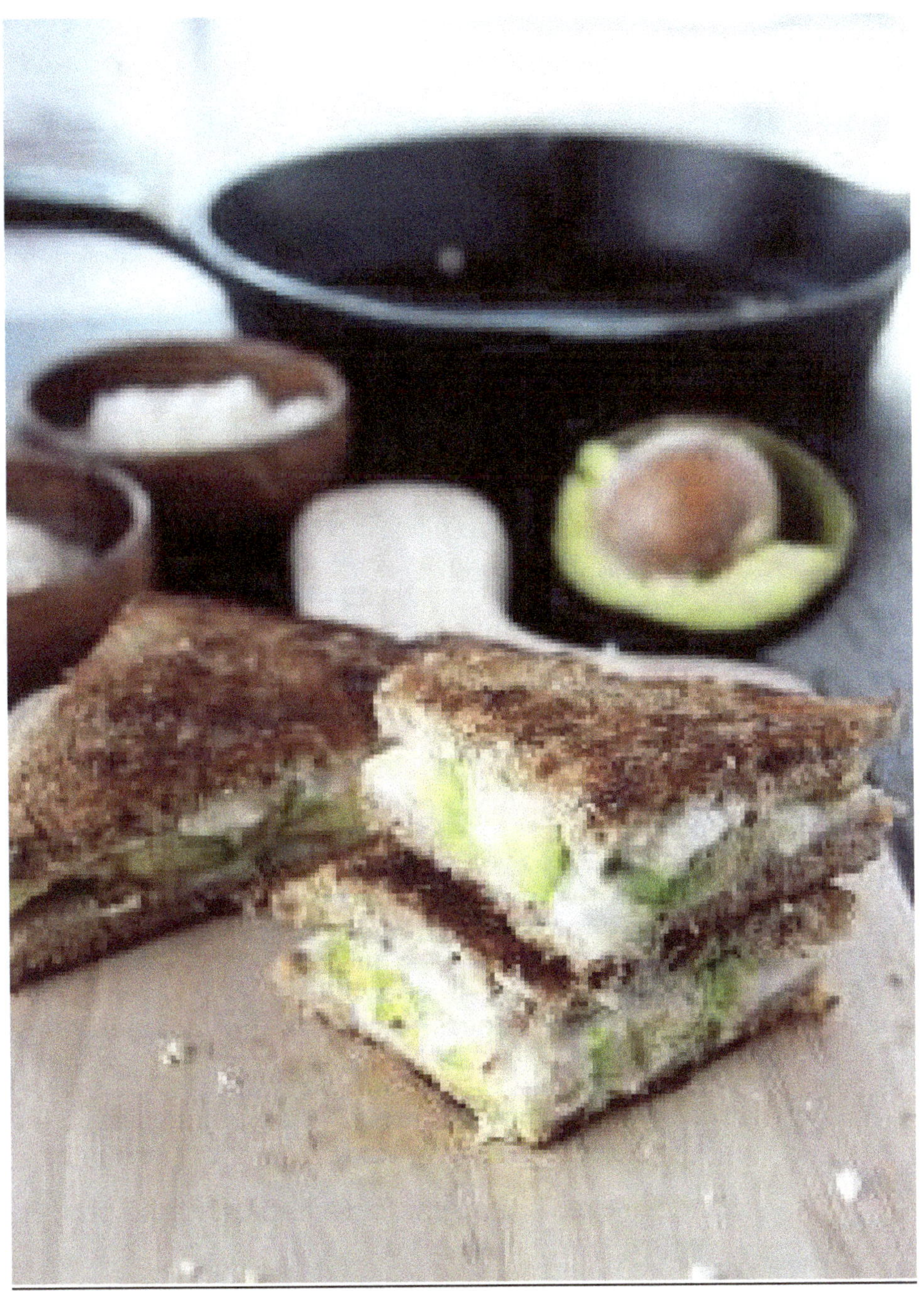

<u>*Preparation Time*</u> : 10 minutes

<u>*Cooking Time*</u> : 10-15 minutes

<u>*Servings*</u> :4

<u>*Ingredients*</u> :

- 1/2 a red onion
- 2 tablespoons fresh coriander
- 1/4 cup cherry tomatoes
- 1/2 a red bell pepper
- 1 tablespoon dulse flakes
- Juice of lime
- Salt to taste
- 3 tablespoons olive oil
- 2 tablespoons tahini
- 1 cup warm chickpeas

<u>*Directions*</u> :

1. Prepare your Air Fryer cooking basket
2. Add chickpeas to your cooking container and cook for 10-15 minutes, making a point to continue blending them every once in a while, until they are altogether warmed
3. Add warmed chickpeas to a bowl and include tahini, salt, lime
4. Utilize a fork to pound chickpeas and fixings in a glue until smooth
5. Include hacked onion, cherry tomatoes, ringer pepper, dulse drops, and olive oil

6. Blend well until consolidated

7. Serve hummus with a couple of cuts of spelt bread

Nutrition : Calories: 95 kcal; Carbohydrates: 5 g; Fat: 5 g; Protein: 5 g

Respiratory Support Tea

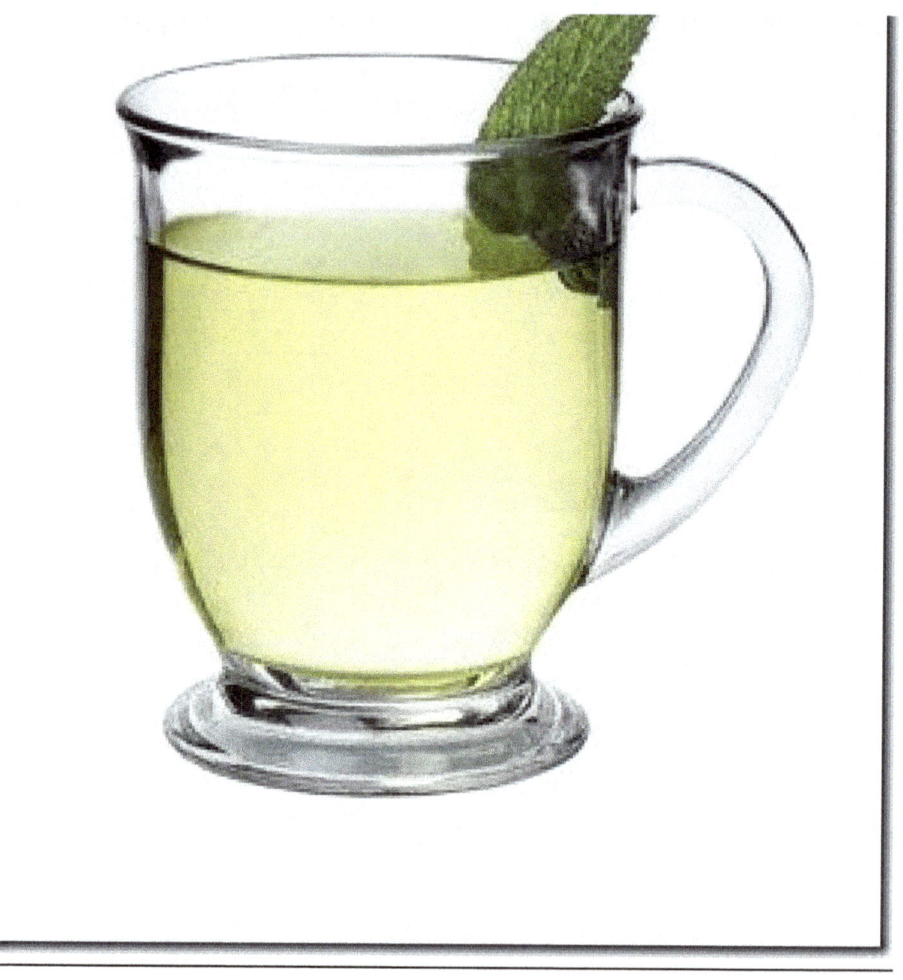

Preparation Time : 5 minutes

Cooking Time : 18 minutes

Servings : 4

Ingredients :

- Rosehip, 2 parts

- Lemon balm, 1 part

- Coltsfoot leaves, 1 part

- Mullein, 1 part

- Osha root, 1 part

- Marshmallow root, 1 part

Directions :

1. Place three cups of water into a pot. Place the Osha root and marshmallow root into the pot. Allow to boil. Let this simmer for ten minutes

2. Now put the remaining Ingredients into the pot and let this steep another eight minutes. Strain.

3. Drink four cups of this tea each day.

4. It's almost that time of year again when everyone is suffering from the dreaded cold. Then that cold turns into a nasty lingering cough. Having these Ingredients on hand will help you be able to get ahead of this year's cold season. When you buy your ingredient, they need to be stored in glass jars. The roots and leaves need to be put into separate jars. You can drink this tea at any time, but it is great for when you need some extra respiratory support.

Nutrition : Calories 35; Sugar 3.4g; Protein 2.3g; Fat 1.5g

Thyme and Lemon Tea

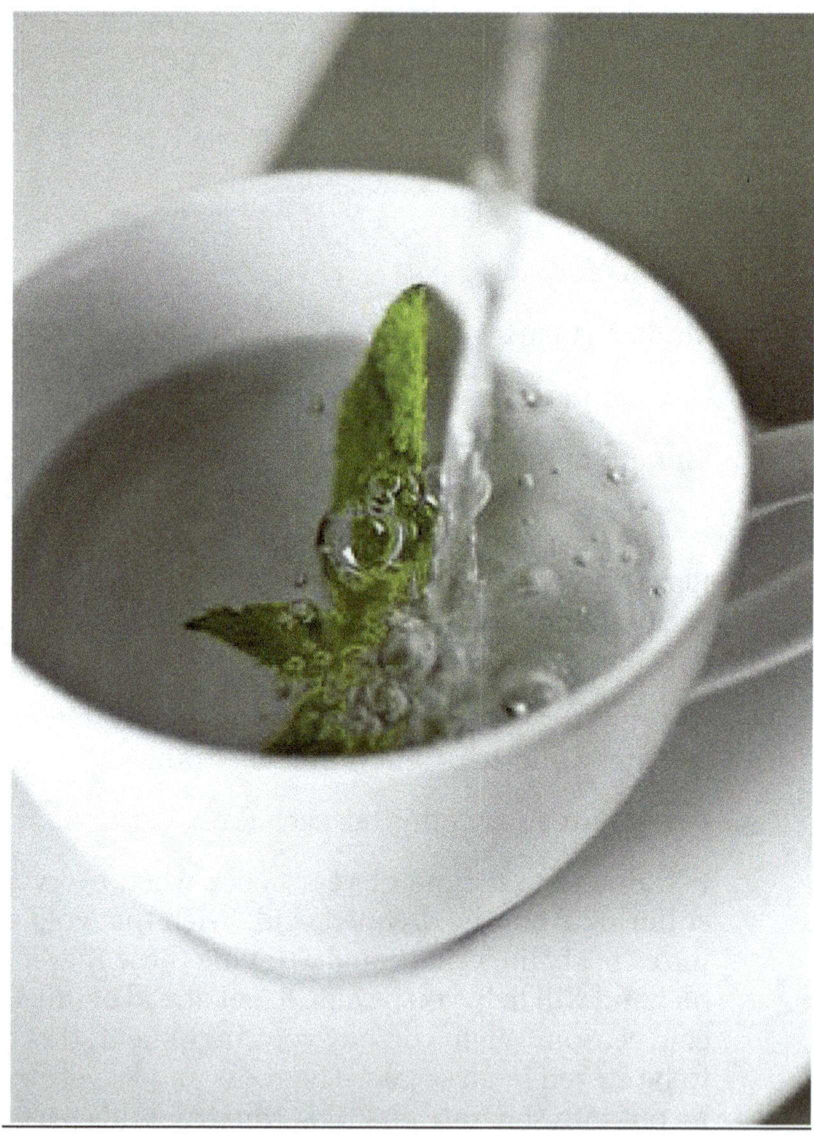

Preparation Time : 5 minutes

Cooking Time : 10 minutes

Servings : 2

Ingredients :

- Key lime juice, 2 tsp.

- Fresh thyme sprigs, 2

Directions :

1. Place the thyme into a canning jar. Boil enough water to cover the thyme sprigs. Cover the jar with a lid and leave it alone for ten minutes. Add the key lime juice. Carefully strain into a mug and add some agave nectar if desired.

Nutrition : Calories 22; Sugar 1.4g; Protein 5.3g; Fat 0.6g

Sore Throat Tea

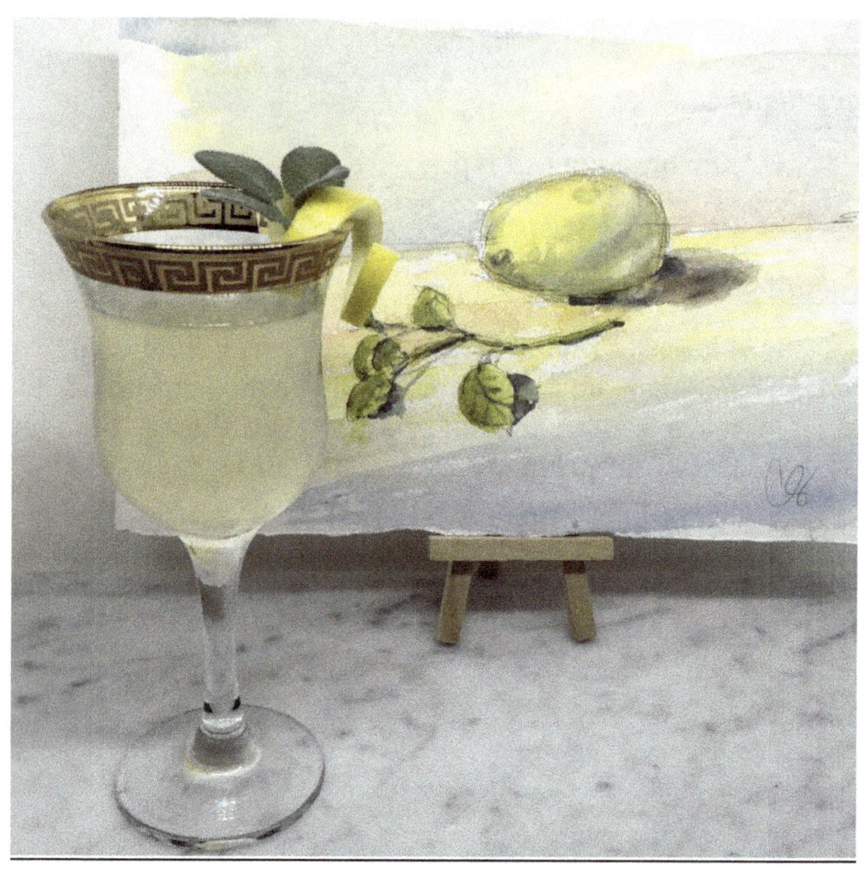

Preparation Time : 8 minutes

Cooking Time : 15 minutes

Servings : 4

Ingredients :

- Sage leaves, 8 to 10 leaves

Directions :

1. Place the sage leaves into a quart canning jar and add water that has boiled until it covers the leaves. Pour the lid on the jar and let sit for 15 minutes.

2. You can use this tea as a gargle to help ease a sore or scratchy throat. Usually, the pain will ease up before you even finish your first cup. This can also be used for inflammations of the throat, tonsils, and mouth since the mucous membranes get soothed by the sage oil. A normal dose would be between three to four cups each day. Every time you take a sip, roll it around in your mouth before swallowing it.

Nutrition : Calories 26; Sugar 2.0g; Protein 7.6g; Fat 3.2g

Autumn Tonic Tea

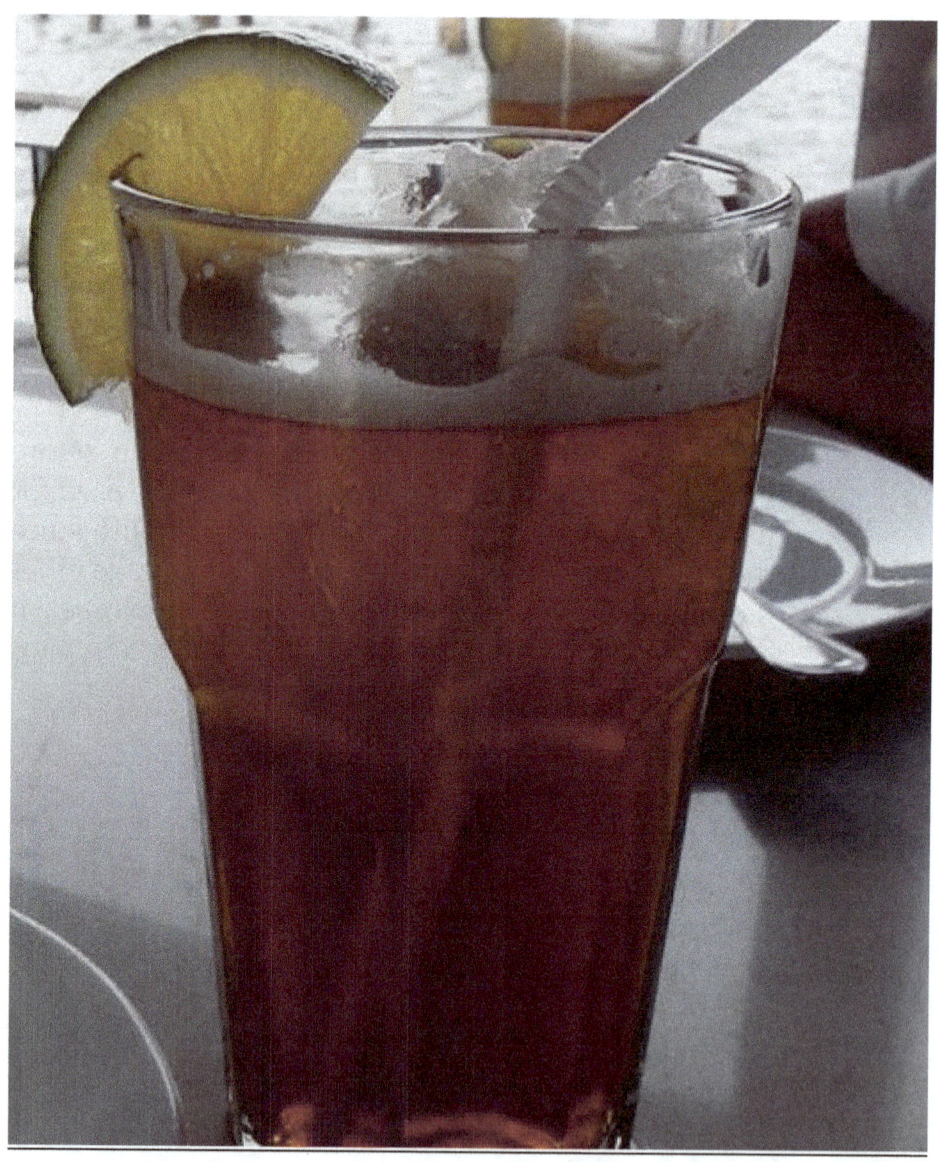

Preparation Time : 10 minutes

Cooking Time : 15 minutes

Servings : 2

Ingredients :

- Dried ginger root, 1 part
- Rosehip, 1 part
- Red clover, 2 parts
- Dandelion root and leaf, 2 parts
- Mullein leaf, 2 parts
- Lemon balm, 3 parts
- Nettle leaf, 4 parts

Directions :

1. Place all of these Ingredients above into a bowl. Stir everything together to mix well. Put into a glass jar with a lid and keep it in a dry place that stays cool.

2. When you want a cup of tea, place four cups of water into a pot. Let this come to a full rolling boil. Place the desired amount of tea blend into a tea strainer, ball, or bag and cover with boiling water. Let sit for 15 minutes. Strain out the herbs and drink it either cold or hot. If you like your tea sweet, add some agave syrup or date sugar.

Nutrition : Calories 43; Sugar 3.8g; Protein 6.5g; Fat 3.9g

Adrenal and Stress Health

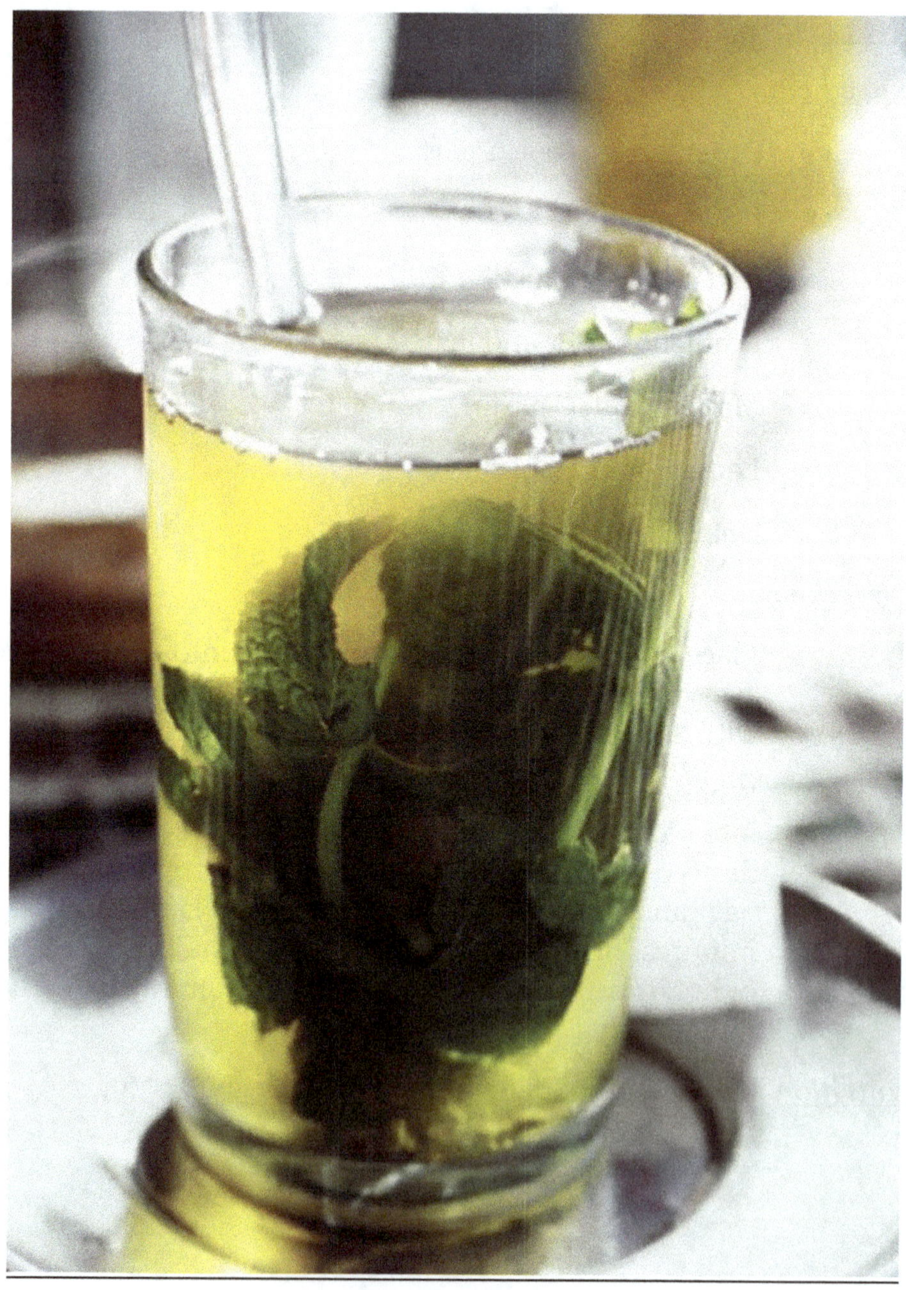

Preparation Time : 12 minutes

Cooking Time : 20 minutes

Servings : 2

Ingredients :

- Bladder wrack, .5 c
- Tulsi holy basil, 1 c
- Shatavari root, 1 c
- Ashwagandha root, 1 c

Directions :

1. Place these Ingredients into a bowl. Stir well to combine.

2. Place mixture in a glass jar with a lid and store in a dry place that stays cool.

3. When you want a cup of tea, place two tablespoons of the tea mixture into a medium pot. Pour in two cups of water. Let this come to a full rolling boil. Turn down heat. Let this simmer 20 minutes. Strain well. If you prefer your tea sweet, you can add some agave syrup or date sugar.

Nutrition : Calories 43; Sugar 2.2g; Protein 4.1g; Fat 2.3g

Lavender Tea

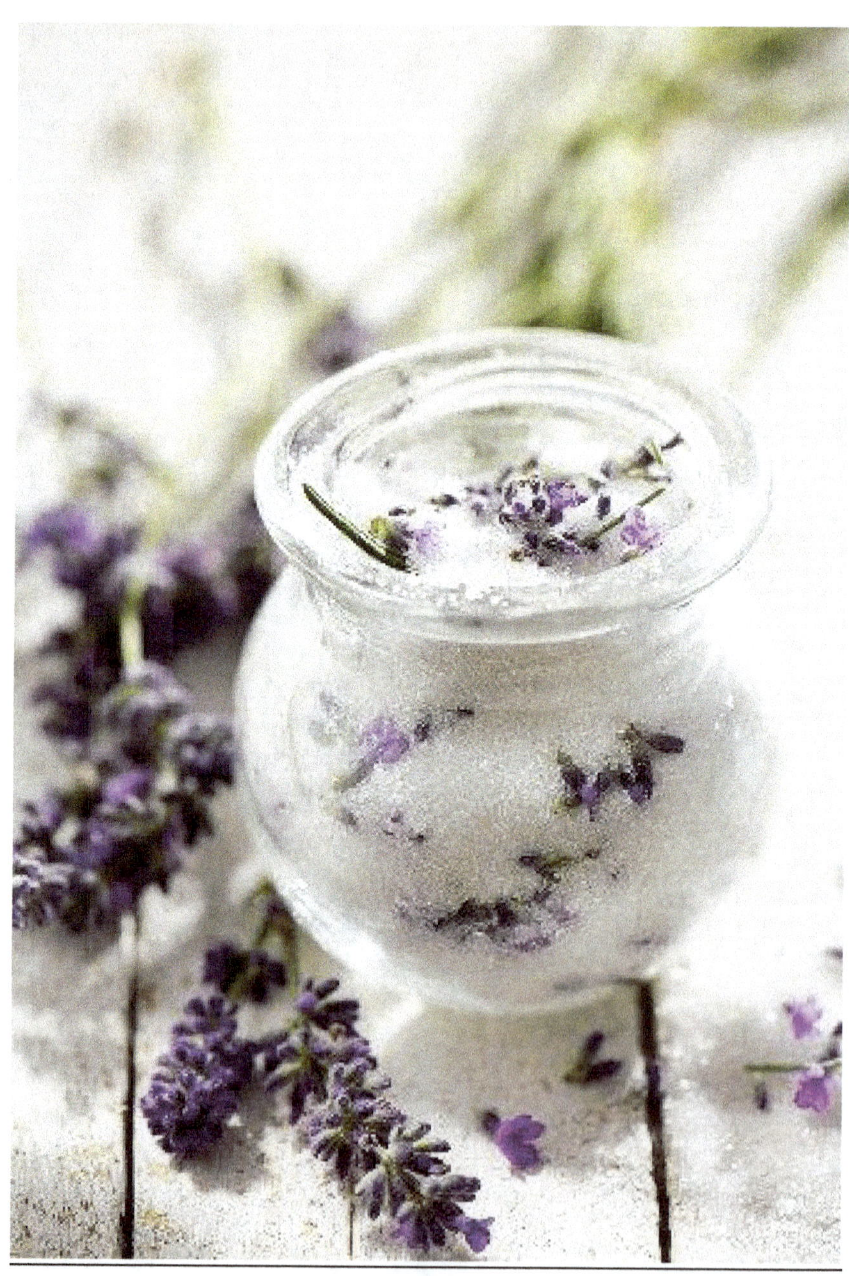

Preparation Time : 5 minutes

Cooking Time : 15 minutes

Servings : 2

Ingredients :

- Agave syrup, to taste

- Dried lavender flowers, 2 tbsp.

- Fresh lemon balm, handful

- Water, 3 c

Directions :

1. Pour the water in a pot and allow to boil.

2. Pour over the lavender and lemon balm. Cover and let sit for five minutes.

3. Strain well. If you prefer your tea sweet, add some agave syrup.

Nutrition : Calories 59; Sugar 6.8g; Protein 3.3g; Fat 1.6g

Fresh Tuna Salad

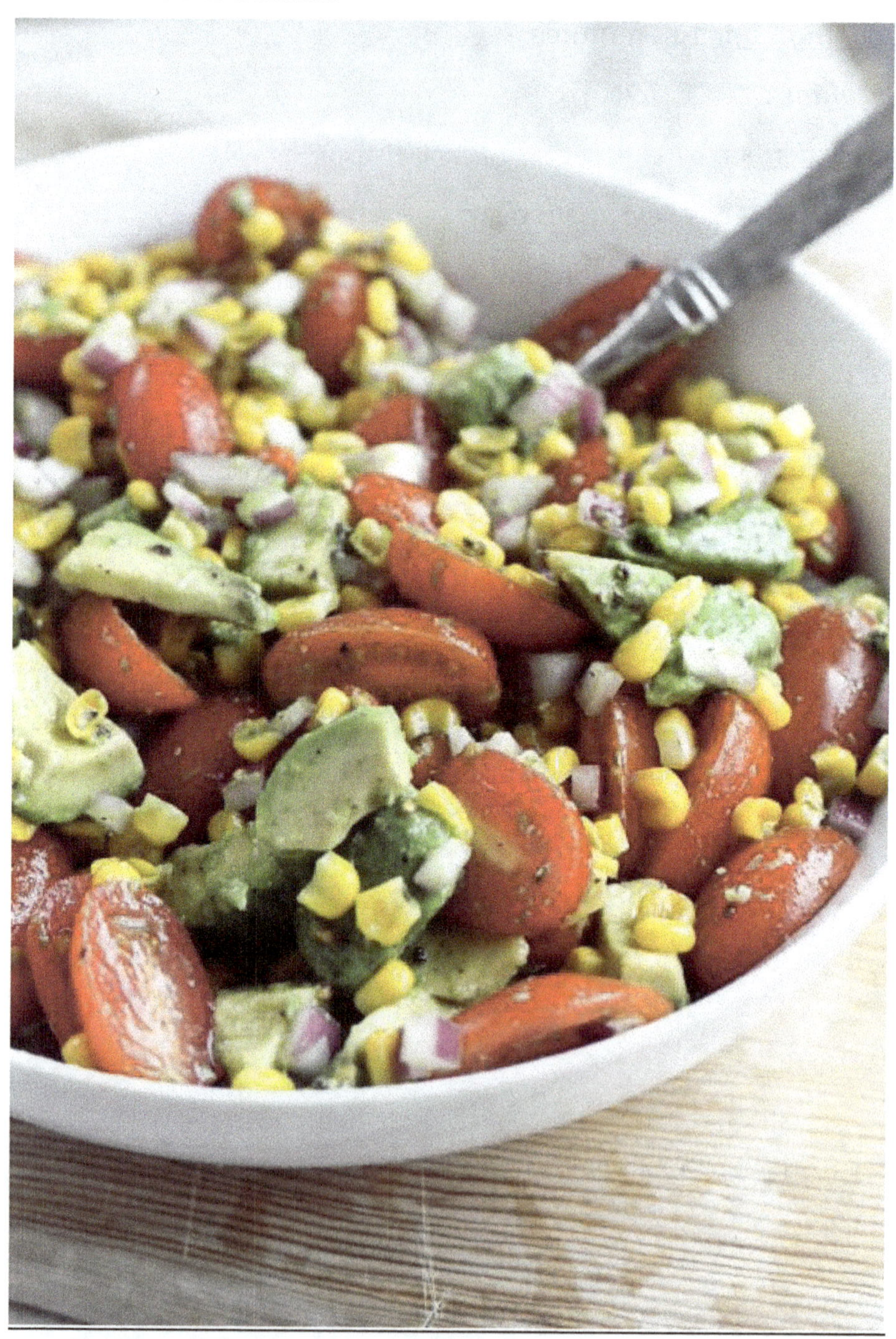

<u>*Preparation Time*</u> : 10 minutes

<u>*Cooking Time*</u> : none

<u>*Servings*</u> : 3

<u>*Ingredients*</u> :

- 1 can tuna (6 oz.)
- 1/3 cup fresh cucumber, chopped
- 1/3 cup fresh tomato, chopped
- 1/3 cup avocado, chopped
- 1/3 cup celery, chopped
- 2 garlic cloves, minced
- 4 tsp. olive oil
- 2 tbsp. lime juice
- Pinch of black pepper

<u>*Directions*</u> :

1. Prepare the dressing by combining olive oil, lime juice, minced garlic and black pepper.
2. Mix the salad ingredients in a salad bowl and drizzle with the dressing.

<u>*Nutrition*</u> : Carbohydrates: 4.8 g Protein: 14.3 g Total sugars: 1.1 g Calories: 212 g

Roasted Portobello Salad

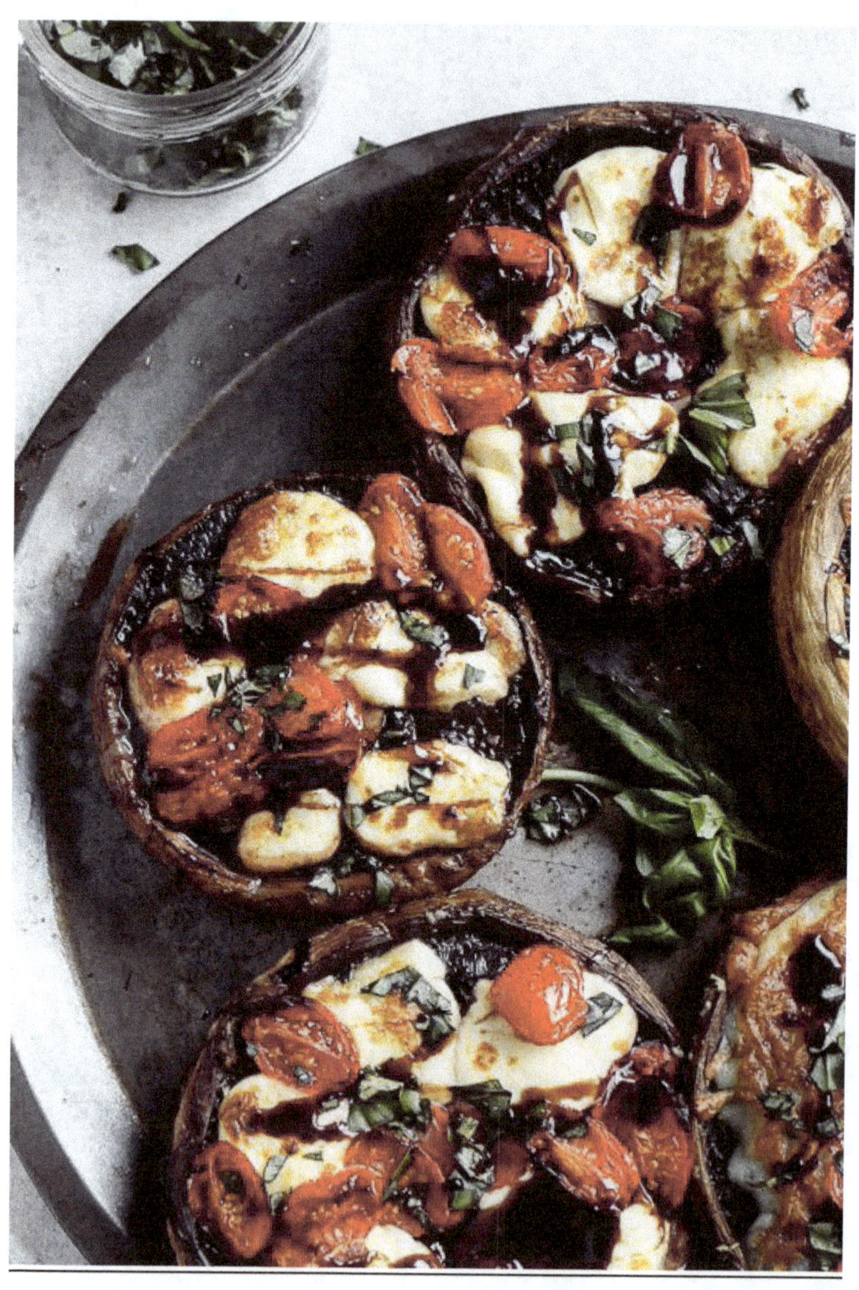

Preparation Time : 10 minutes

Cooking Time : none

Servings : 4

Ingredients :

- 11/2 lb. Portobello mushrooms, stems trimmed
- 3 heads Belgian endive, sliced
- 1 small red onion, sliced
- 4 oz. blue cheese
- 8 oz. mixed salad greens
- Dressing:
- 3 tbsp. red wine vinegar
- 1 tbsp. Dijon mustard
- 2/3 cup olive oil
- Salt and pepper to taste

Directions :

1. Preheat the oven to 450F.
2. Prepare the dressing by whisking together vinegar, mustard, salt and pepper. Slowly add olive oil while whisking.
3. Cut the mushrooms and arrange them on a baking sheet, stem-side up. Coat the mushrooms with some dressing and bake for 15 minutes.
4. In a salad bowl toss the salad greens with onion, endive and cheese. Sprinkle with the dressing.
5. Add mushrooms to the salad bowl.

<u>*Nutrition*</u> : Carbohydrates: 22.3 g; Protein: 14.9 g; Total sugars: 2.1 g; Calories: 501

Greek Salad

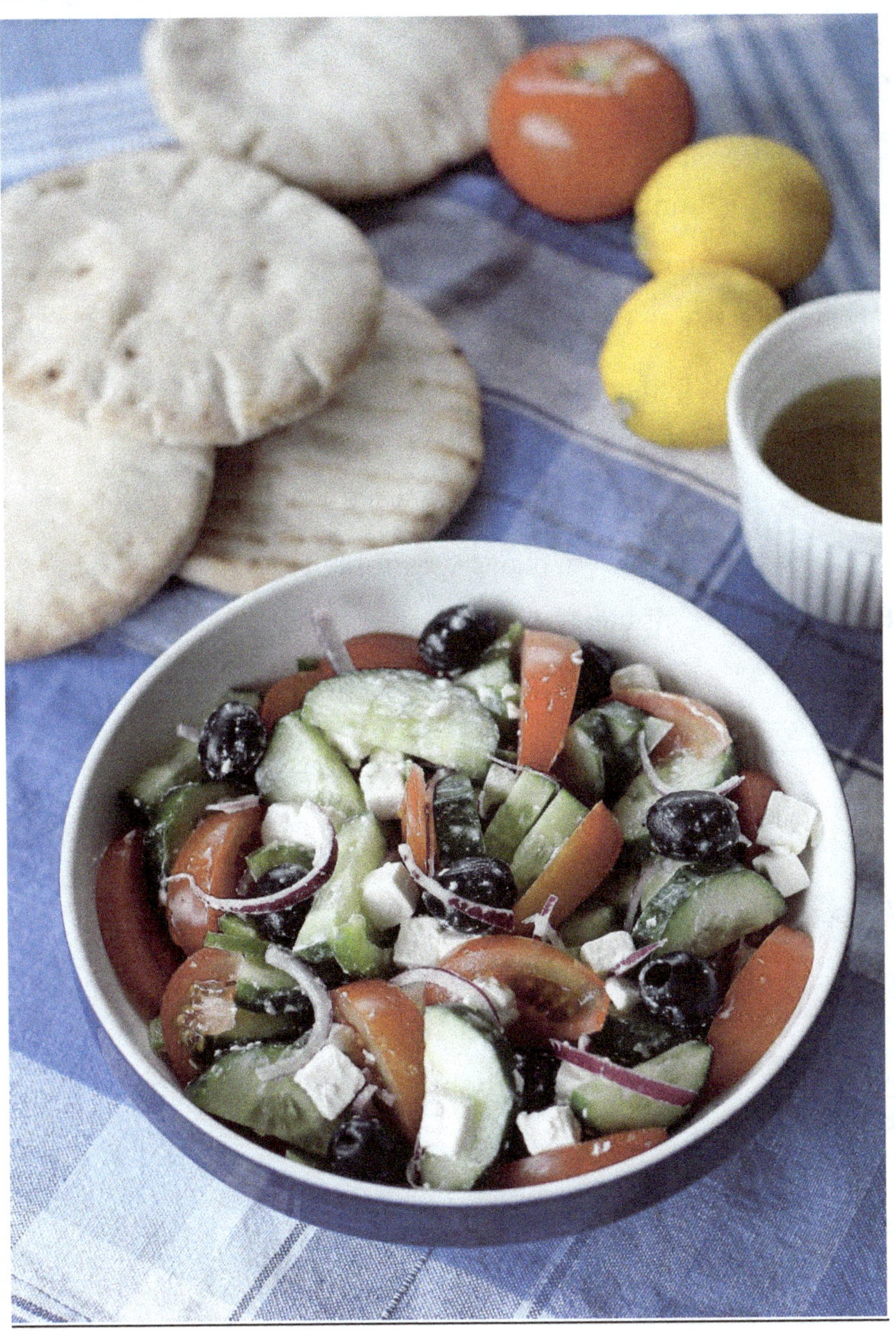

<u>*Preparation Time*</u> : 10 minutes

<u>*Cooking Time*</u> : 0 minutes

<u>*Servings*</u> : 1-2

<u>*Ingredients*</u> :

- 1 Romaine head, torn in bits
- 1 cucumber sliced
- 1 pint cherry tomatoes, halved
- 1 green pepper, thinly sliced
- 1 onion sliced into rings
- 1 cup kalamata olives
- 1 ½ cups feta cheese, crumbled

For dressing combine:

- 1 cup olive oil
- 1/4 cup lemon juice
- 2 tsp. oregano
- Salt and pepper

<u>*Directions*</u> :

1. Lay Ingredients on plate.
2. Drizzle dressing over salad

<u>*Nutrition*</u> : Calories: 107; Carbohydrates: 18g; Fat: 1.2 g; Protein: 1g

Alkaline Spring Salad

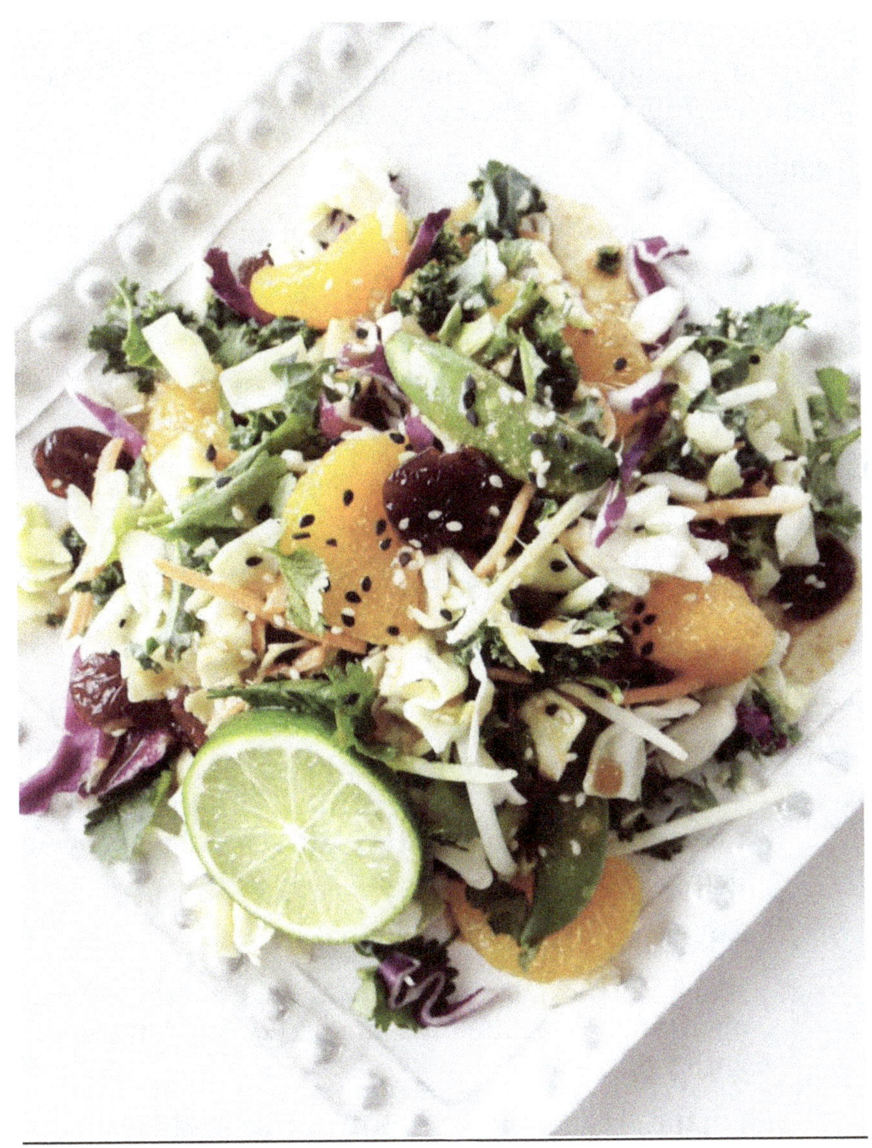

Preparation Time : 10 minutes

Cooking Time : 0 minutes

Servings : 1-2

Eating seasonal fruits and vegetables is a fabulous way of taking care of yourself and the environment at the same time. This alkaline-electric salad is delicious and nutritious.

Ingredients :

- 4 cups seasonal approved greens of your choice
- 1 cup cherry tomatoes
- 1/4 cup walnuts
- 1/4 cup approved herbs of your choice

For the dressing:

- 3-4 key limes
- 1 tbsp. of homemade raw sesame
- Sea salt and cayenne pepper

Directions :

1. First, get the juice of the key limes. In a small bowl, whisk together the key lime juice with the homemade raw sesame "tahini" butter. Add sea salt and cayenne pepper, to taste.

2. Cut the cherry tomatoes in half.

3. In a large bowl, combine the greens, cherry tomatoes, and herbs. Pour the dressing on top and "massage" with your hands.

4. Let the greens soak up the dressing. Add more sea salt, cayenne pepper, and herbs on top if you wish. Enjoy!

<u>*Nutrition*</u> : Calories: 77; Carbohydrates: 11g